TOTALLY BLADDERED

The true story of an
illogical urological nightmare

JACQ EMKES

Copyright © 2021 Jacq Emkes
Print Edition

Written by JACQUELINE EMKES
Cover Design by Kostis Pavlou 99Designs
Cartoons by Nick Newman
Illustrations by Jacqueline Emkes using eLearningheroes

All rights reserved. No part of this publication may be reproduced, distributed or transmitted in any form or by any means, or stored in a database or retrieval system, without the prior written permission of the publisher.

Disclaimer: The material in this book is for mature audiences only and contains graphic content. It is intended only for those aged 18 and older.

Contents

Dedication	v
Foreword by Jerome	vii
Prologue	1
1. Hello from Kidney World, 11 November 2010	9
2. Bellini breakfast, Tue, 02 Feb 2016	100
3. Bladder and brain still not in unison	101
4. House of Cards, Sat, 16 Apr 2016	102
5. NICE Guidelines	104
6. Auf Wiedersehen, Thu, 21 Apr 2016	105
7. Open for business 24/7, Sat, 07 May 2016	109
8. On it like a car bonnet, Sun, 15 May 2016	110
9. I'll try not to kill you this week, Mon, 30 May 2016	112
10. Whitehall, Sat, 04 Jun 2016	114
11. Paper curtains with the fabulous Melanie Reid, Sun, 05 Jun 2016	115
12. Stormy weather, Sat, 11 Jun 2016	116
13. M.B.E. Motivational Brave Educational Melanie Reid, June 2016	119
14. Bugoff Oneoff, Wed, 14 Sep 2016	121
15. Bladder Buddy, Sat, 24 Sep 2016	123
16. Trolley Dolly, Sat, 12 Nov 2016 another hospital stays	126
17. Absolute Dogs Bollocks, Sat, 03 Dec 2016	127
18. Why are you Here, Mon, 30 Nov	129
19. Squashed bananas, Sat, 10 Dec 2016	130
20. Mice and men, Fri, 16 Dec 2016	131
21. Cakes at Christmas Long Live the NHS	132
22. Patients, virtue and patience, Mon, 27 Feb 2017	134
23. Pacing, Gin and Caffeine, Wed, 01 Mar 2017	136
24. What a laugh, Wed, 12 Apr 2017	137
25. Piddles make puddles, Sun, 23 Apr 2017	138
26. Hippo, Cock and Bull Story, Fri, 19 May 2017	144

27. Prosecco, Sat, 03 Jun 2017	147
28. Marbles … lost my, Sat, 10 Jun 2017	150
29. Bonkers, Sun, 02 Jul 2017	152
30. Dragon Tattoo, Tue, 22 Aug 2017	156
31. Shaggy Dog, Mon, 11 Sep 2017	158
32. Royal College of Testicles, Fri, 15 Sep 2017	160
33. On the wrong platform, Sun, 24 Sep 2017	162
34. BAPS, Wed, 27 Sep 2017	164
35. NHS hospital Wednesday, Wed, 27 Sep 2017	167
36. Stopcock, Sun, 08 Oct 2017	168
37. One flew over the cuckoo's nest, Fri, 13 Oct 2017	169
38. Ophelia Week, Sat, 21 Oct 2017	171
39. Ophelia part 2, Thu, 26 Oct 2017	172
40. Ophelia part 3 – the clinicians, Thu, 26 Oct 2017	175
41. Fireworks, Mon, 30 Nov	177
42. The English Patients, Sun, 12 Nov 2017	179
43. Piddle and Patsy, Sun, 19 Nov 2017	183
44. Jam pots, Sat, 25 Nov 2017	185
45. Hallelujah, Sat, 16 Dec 2017	187
46. A landmark step in local GP services! Wed, 03 Jan 2018	189
47. Bingo, Thu, 11 Jan 2018	192
48. Uncle to the rescue, Wed, 17 Jan 2018	194
49 Chocolate, Sat, 20 Jan 2018	195
50. Nice waiting rooms, Sun, 28 Jan 2018	196
51. Waiting Room part 2, Tue, 30 Jan 2018	198
52. Naked surgeon, Sat, 03 Feb 2018	199
53. Fri, 09 Feb 2018 Willy Wonka	200
54. Minority Report or bionic robotics, Tue, 20 Feb 2018	203
55. Bilbo Baggins, Thu, 22 Feb 2018	204
56. Farted and left the room, Thu, 01 Mar 2018	205
57. Tough. Shit. Thu, 29 Mar 2018	209
58. The first decade	212
About the Author	223

Dedication

For Oliver Rory and Heidi – Gaggsie!

For all those coping with 'bladderations'. I had no idea until I joined you.

Massive thanks to my ever awesome family, my husband Daniel, my children and their partners. You are incredible. Thank you to my brother Mike and all my friends. Always there, always ready to make things alright.

Nick wow such fabulous cartoons and friendship, thank you.

How could I ever have managed without the legend that is Jerome. Thank you so much for sorting everything and making me laugh.

Foreword by Jerome

I was asked to perform operation fifteen for Jacqueline Emkes just over a decade ago and am delighted to write this preface to her book based on a series of blogs that have proved to be a cathartic reflection of her healthcare journey balancing medical issues, work life as a secondary school mathematics teacher, home and family life, as well as being a campaigner for bladder / continence health in the House of Commons committees.

Her journey had started three years before we met, and has continued as a vicious circle of one intervention after another, each aiming to solve one problem but with knock-on effects that mean more consultations, opinions and operations are needed. Her account shows how medical and surgical complexity builds slowly at first and then more rapidly, like an exponential graph that she would be familiar with in a maths class. This led to the analogy of being a "frequent flier", a theme that runs through the book, but clearly with less rewards for being a patient compared with the benefits in the travel industry.

Some of the operations Jacq has undergone have been minor (like a short flight) but many have been major (unquestionably "long haul"), and with a destination ("cure") that remains tantalisingly elusive. In medicine, it is important to recognise that simple and straightforward acute conditions can be fixed (a broken arm, for example) but longstanding, complex "chronic" conditions cannot be cured (otherwise they would have been already) but have to be managed and lived with. It was during discussions about this, and the need to manage expectations that the comment "I cannot cure you but can make you laugh" first arose as a combination of Voltaire's quote *"The art of medicine consists of amusing the patient while nature cures the disease"* the old adage that *"laughter is the best medicine"*.

The parallels between flights and operations allow Jacq to compare nurses to air stewards, and surgeons to pilots, and departure lounges to medical waiting rooms, as well as delays for appointments to flight cancellations that are always disappointing and frustrating and even economy class on a normal ward to an "upgrade" to first class on an Intensive Care Unit. Complications during the treatment, such as the problems she has had with allergies, are therefore the equivalent to turbulence during a flight. She also explains that, when the operation is over, the sense of being "on your own" without "in flight support" can leave you feeling vulnerable despite the euphoria of sleeping in your own bed and eating your own food.

Jacq uses her experience and knowledge of the system to offer advice to other patients, from unexplained observations that it always six weeks for a follow up appointment, to the fact that curtains on wards are not soundproof, and conversations in waiting rooms certainly are not private – if nothing else, I doubt anyone will ever book a holiday from a waiting room again!

There are serious messages too, including regarding consent, where percentage risks of complications may not be immediately meaningful. Translating these risks into personal circumstances, and perhaps even more so of personal consequence would fit the modernisation of obtaining consent, with the Montgomery ruling. Unlike in 2009, for Jacq's first operation, current practice should be that "informed consent" represents a series of discussions, and that the paperwork, which is actually the least part of the process, should be completed in advance of the day of surgery, and countersigned as "final confirmation" in much the same way that the flight plan of an aeroplane is all planned in advance, with the final checks before taking to the runway simply to make sure that everything that has been planned and agreed is correct and in place.

Jacq recognises that this takes a lot of time, both for the patient and the clinician, and it is not clear where this time will come from in a system of cancelled and rearranged appointments…

There is wisdom and many insights into a health system that is under pressure for service providers to reflect on too. Broken urodynamics machines, team shortages, malfunctioning nerve stimulators a whole new alphabet of acronyms, delayed results mid-stream urine samples(msu) for urinary tract infections (uti), forgotten allergies, rescheduled appointments and last-minute cancellations, delayed surgeons, and a pet puppy "admitted within minutes" but her father "on a trolley for hours".

Despite these challenges, patients continue to expect that their clinicians have all the information (if not all the answers as well) and therefore understandably find questions like "what is the purpose of this appointment" disconcerting. To maintain the aeronautical analogy, this would be like hearing the pilot ask the passengers where they were flying to.

The book covers the frustration of the patient having to explain that they are not right, or why they feel that they are not, or repeating the background history again and again to people who the patient believes should already know this important information. In this respect, we constantly hear "it should all be in my notes" and have to explain the painful truth that often it is not, as there may not be an established method to share that information, and even if it is available, it can be difficult to access, including for there to be enough time before a consultation to find and read it all, particularly in complex patients, where, by definition, there is more information from more sources. Indeed, for patients with Chronic conditions Jacq emphasises the need to "empower the patient" recommending that results are given directly to the patient because they usually know what should be done with them and about them. In agreement with this, there is a drive that all communication should be directed primarily to the patient and copied to the GP and other clinicians, rather than the traditional approach the other way around.

Over the course of her book, Jacq has downloaded her experience of her health and healthcare like downloading the content of her own medical "black box" in-flight recorder. This represents fifteen years acquired knowledge wisdom and insight to help others negotiate a complex system, and to remember that each patient is a person, and has a life and a family that their condition needs to be treated in conjunction with, and for which a team approach is essential – hence the "three men in a boat" for the key players travelling in conjunction with Jacq throughout her story, including my part of *"Putting the logical into urological"*.

Being unwell needs a great deal of personal resolve, and this book shows how Jacq has battled with her bladder, back and breathing, and has done so against the odds, and with a well maintained sense of humour. I never expected my quip *"I cannot cure you but can make you laugh"* to appear in cartoon form on the front of a book, and am sorry that it has not been possible to cure you, but we have certainly enjoyed a lot of laughter on the journey, and I am sure that the readers of your book will share the funny side with you.

Jerome
October 2021

THE STORY ABOUT THE DAYS, MONTHS AND YEARS AFTER AN ACCIDENT TO MY BLADDER

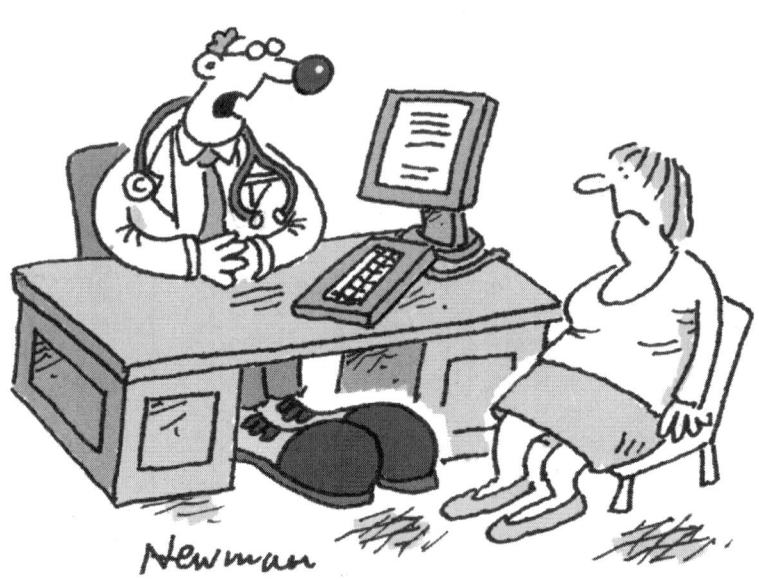

Prologue

The beginning of 2009 saw historic snow falls. The summer was historically hot! Minister and MP expenses scandals raged. Swine flu 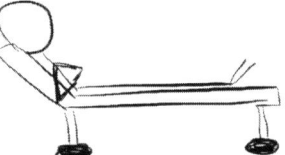 was prevalent in the UK brought in from Mexico. Talk of a pandemic was rumoured but did not materialise. As for me, I was a full-time teacher of maths at a secondary school near home. My 4 teenage children were moving on through GCSEs and A Levels and as a celebration I took the girls to Paris to celebrate the end of exams. I too had just handed in my Masters. How on earth I got that done I have no idea. Paris from our nearest London station St Pancras, was a total relax, giggling and chattering with my daughters. On my return I made myself a long overdue GP appointment. I had struggled to control the effects of fibroids and ovarian cysts. These, as many women will testify, are horrendous. Not least because of unexpected bleeding, as in flooding. For weeks on end. It can happen without any warning. Awkward for work, social life and sport. Having tried to use hormone therapy and various medications my gp suggested I see the local gynaecologist team. She asked me who I would like to make an appointment with. Having not a clue, I accepted her suggested surgeon. The appointment was duly organised. Tests, scans and consultations were made. It was decided that she would try a procedure known as an ablation. This was to cauterise the areas causing so much bleeding. It would be a day case and not likely to cause any issues. Coming round from anaesthesia the surgeon explained it had not worked. discharged home a few hours later, I collapsed on my bathroom floor. Rushed into hospital with heavy bleeding the consultant was again available, sympathetic and very concerned. It was now necessary for a hysterectomy as soon as possible.

The hysterectomy was hastily arranged, booked, pre assessed and time off work scheduled. I was so embarrassed to ask for 6 weeks at the beginning of the school year. Minutes before being wheeled into the operation I signed the consent form. Relieved to be finally going for it. That consent form was set to haunt me in later years.

The operation itself seemed to go well. The recovery in the hospital took about 5 days and then I was discharged home. There followed problems. I seemed to have continuous bladder infections requiring antibiotics. I needed painkillers for right sided pain. Bruising around my abdomen was so extensive; it spread to my back and upper legs too. By Week 6 and my follow up appointment I was desperate to get back to work.

Pre 2009

My husband and I met whilst training to be Chartered Accountants in 1982. We lived and worked in London and after our wedding in 1986 we 'settled down'. Well no. Daniel joined his father's family tea business and travelled the world. I stayed in South London and raised our children. We moved to Bedford in 2001. The children were all happy at school and I retrained as a secondary maths teacher at a school. By 2004 I was fully installed in a North Bedford school, teaching maths, accounting and then to my infinite surprise gained my master's at Cambridge. I had to pinch myself. Was this really me? I loved the students, my colleagues and running and skiing and Cornwall. Life was brilliant.

As anyone having had an operation will know, doctors tell you it will be 6 weeks for recovery. It is always 6 weeks! Why 6 weeks? God only knows. But 6 it is. At my week 6 follow up, I was declared fit for phased return to work and discharged from gynaecology clinic.

Subsequent physiotherapy appointments proved difficult on account of extreme pain down my right side. The physiotherapist was concerned and spoke to the consultant directly. In due course a CT[1] was arranged. It was now December 2009.

The CT was on a Thursday afternoon. I organised lesson plans and homework for the colleagues taking my class. The CT was fine. I consented for injection of dye known as contrast, which I understood would give a better image. Again, I had no idea what I was consenting! But, several hours later, at home. I began to itch, and burn, and wheeze and collapse once more. Emergency treatment at hospital and then days later I discovered I had had an anaphylactic reaction to the CT contrast dye. However, good news, the consultant rang me to tell me

---

[1] A CT is computed tomography scan which combines lots of xrays which are computer-processed to show what it looks like inside.

the CT showed all was 'normal' recovery after hysterectomy. By February 2010, pain and infections were ever worsening and my physiotherapist had sent my CT disc to her friend, a London Consultant Urologist whom I later named Wingrave, to review the CT of December. Alas in a phone call I was told London had reviewed the imaging and, in their opinion, my right ureter was obstructed. That is, the pipework taking urine from kidney to bladder. They advised an urgent MRI. Once more I arranged cover with my head of department at school. The radiographer was lovely, kind, chatty. The MRI seemed to take forever. Then, I was asked to move to the ultrasound room for further imaging. My thoughts still 'in school' I said I could not possibly wait to see the consultant who was 'held up' in surgery. Off I rushed to school. I did detention duty, taught observed lessons and sailed through a lesson I had designed for a job interview practice. I was living on adrenaline. Flying through the day until a wonderful colleague found me to say I looked a bit shocked. Was I ok? Of course. I spoke. But then explained. Without further ado she made me go home and await the consultants' call.

That call really was the end of life as I knew it. The consultant sent me straight back into the hospital that very night. It is a very strange thing, finally, somehow acknowledging I was in trouble, I accepted morphine and tried to sleep. Of course, the morphine set my bladder into retention. In retention the pain worsened. I accepted more morphine. But still my bladder filled and was not draining. By morning a Consultant Mr Urologist arrived. He looked at the images and decided there were stones in my right kidney and that he could see obstruction of my right ureter. And retention of my bladder. An indwelling catheter was urgently requested He proposed he would operate immediately. Hours later he rang the ward phone, to tell me the operation had been cancelled. Did we have health insurance? Vaguely aware that my husband's office maybe did, we rang the insurers. Indeed, we were covered. In a bizarre change of plan, we had to persuade the ward staff to let me leave the safety of 'NHS-land', still attached to drips and bits. They were not happy; it was against the rules. But after all it was the surgeon who had suggested it. Daniel after some extensive searching found a wheelchair. Wrapped in borrowed blankets to hide the drips, somehow, we got to the car, drove across town to private hospital land. There awaited a whole operating team and Mr Urologist too. The relief at finally being sorted overcame the very strange change of location! The operation was declared a success. He 'lost' the stones, found resistance in the ureter and so inserted what is known as a stent.[2] The immediate relief was fantastic. All that fluid could now drain to the bladder from the kidney. Indeed, from bladder to leg bag too. Euphoria set in and I was cured. Hurrah.

So well did I feel I agreed to an interview for a new job the following week.

---

[2] A Stent: A sort of hollow wire which hooks into the kidney and then leads down to the bladder where it is anchored.

I went. I got the job. I felt amazing. Alas only 2 weeks later, infections had taken a hold once more, the stents were encrusted and removed only to be replaced in another operation in March 2010. This pattern was repeated, and the story continued in a blog I started shortly thereafter. I never did start my new job properly. I was never fit enough to teach full time again. The support, understanding and empathy of the staff at my old and new schools never ceases to amaze me. I had, overnight, become, a Statutory Sick Pay, Occupational Health, phased returner nightmare. All because, during that fateful hysterectomy operation the surgeon had injured my right ureter.

Summer 2010

In the summer of 2010, I underwent major surgery in Bedford. Mr Urologist opened up my abdomen in a 'hockey stick'[3] incision. Once open he could see the build-up of fluid in my right ureter. This ureter he cut, split the top of my bladder to form a tube, known as a Boari flap[4] and fashioned that to the remaining stub of ureter. Inserting stents[5], indwelling catheters[6] and

---

[3] A hockey stick incision is a cut down the side of the abdomen then across in a J or hockey stick shape!
[4] Boari Flap Drainage is re-established by re-implanting the ureter into the bladder, by fashioning a tube of bladder to reach up to the ureter above the blockage (a bladder flap).
[5] Stents A ureteral stent is a thin tube that's placed in your ureter to help drain urine from your kidney. One end of the tube is inside your kidney, and the other end is in your bladder.

maximum pain relief he despatched me back to the ward. Two weeks later I was home and trying to recover. Alas when the stent was removed in September 2010, the ureter once more collapsed. I was again rushed into hospital for more stents, more operations and the story continued in my blog which I began after the 10th operation.

Trying to distract myself as I lay in a hospital bed. I began to liken my hospital admissions to being on a plane. Seat belt on. Hostess trolley wheeled past. Cabin crew or nurses with the bell. It seemed funny then. Now a decade later, how could I ever have imagined I'd still be writing about the world of medicine, bladders and spines? It is a very private story. If you find it funny that is good. If it is a little too rude and offensive, I am sorry, it is just a moment in time. If it makes you cry and feel pity, then stop that straight away. That is a wasted emotion. Send me a funny joke, a silly story a normal day for a normal body…those are the best. Many of the blogs are based on emails from my surgeon who, for the blog I have named Jerome. He is the one who came up with the idea that all the surgeons could be the men in a boat. He decided that as his name did not begin with J, but everyone else's including mine did, he would adopt the name Jerome as in JKJ. The other doctors I call Dipstick,

---

[6] A catheter is a small tube, made of latex or silicone, that is put into your bladder to allow the urine to drain out. It is put in either through the waterpipe (urethral catheter) or through the lower part of the tummy (suprapubic catheter) • The outside part of the catheter is often connected to a bag, so the bladder is kept empty; the bag is worn on your leg or around your tummy. (https://www.baus.org.uk/_userfiles/pages/files/Patients/Leaflets/Catheter.pdf)

Wingrave and Uncle Montmerency. Hopefully for reasons which will become obvious! I cannot explain why writing this blog somehow helps. But it does. It is an attempt to put the **logical** into the uro**logical**.

1. Hello from Kidney World, 11 November 2010

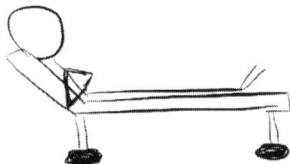

Hello from Kidney World. Well, you will not be surprised to hear that having had a stent out and dilatation of ureter, the 10th operation since September. I ended up back in hospital in total agony. I thenThen endured operation 11, to put yet another new stent in. Mr Urology had referred me to London to see another surgeon. Why ever I had resisted asking for a second opinion.?

The next weeks limped along, Christmas came and went, New Year 2011 arrived, and we went for a ski. Mad I know. But I still thought I was ok. Ski-ing was a bit painful really. But I found I was better if I did not turn on the right side. That made my skiing super-fast. The children were really impressed! The ski lifts were also a bit tricky but straightening my leg across the family and sticking it out the gondola window helped enormously. Much to the consternation of the liftie guys!

FLIGHTS 5 FEBRUARY e story continued in my blog which I began after the 10th operation.

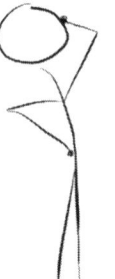 Trying to distract myself as I lay in a hospital bed. I began to liken my hospital admissions to being on a plane. Seat belt on. Hostess trolley wheeled past. Cabin crew or nurses with the bell. It seemed funny then. Now a decade later, how could I ever have imagined I'd still be writing about the world of medicine, bladders and spines? It is a very private story. If you find it funny that is good. If it is a little too rude and offensive, I am sorry, it is just a moment in time. If it makes you cry and feel pity, then stop that straight away. That is a wasted emotion. Send me a funny joke, a silly story a normal day for a normal body…those are the best. Many of the blogs are based on emails from my surgeon who, for the blog I have named Jerome. He is the one who in a final paragraph of a serious and long clinical letter, added the idea that all the surgeons should be the men in a boat. He decided that as his name did not begin with a J, but everyone else's including mine did, he would adopt the name Jerome as in JKJ. The other doctors I call Dipstick, Wingrave and Uncle Montmerency. Hopefully for reasons which will become obvious! I cannot explain why writing this blog somehow helps. But it does. It is an attempt to put the **logical** into the uro**logical**.

January 2011

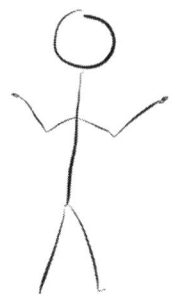
Having been cared for by Mr Urology in my local hospital it became clear my situation was just not improving over the course of 2010. Mr Urology, the surgeon who had tried to put stents in and out plus a massive operation to join the kidney to my bladder, had all seemingly failed. I was therefore referred to see a London specialist. His speciality is women's reconstruction, so I reckoned that made him an ideal person to work out what on earth to do. Not least because he was in fact the friend of my physio. I was now recognised as a frequent flyer in terms of the analogy patients in hospital being similar to passengers on aeroplanes. As on the plane, hospitals give you an individual TV, flat bed (even got remote control on that), nurses like the cabin crew, those trays of meals supplied at strange times 'dinner' at 5:30! No champagne in hospital but of course but marvellous complimentary plug-in cocktails, IV lines of medicines! Pilots like surgeons, and their teams, issued exciting information snippets from time to time. Top in-flight movie? That would have been my blood pressure readings, oxygen levels, temperature. They were all plotted in a superb scatter diagram. This reminded me of my real-life teaching maths in secondary school. In January I was treated in London. This week saw the introduction of new flights aka operations, now taking place from

London. Operation 12 and Operation 13. Or Flight 12 and Flight 13. The blog gained momentum…

Blog entry: 22 January 2011

The ground staff, i.e., a porter, carried my bag to my room explained ubiquitous nurse-call-button, sticky back plastic visitor's chair. I changed into the cotton navy operating gown, dressing gown and hermetically sealed white slippers – all provided in a neat little British Airways type bag. Oh, and white in-flight stockings – individually measured fitted and squeezed on. I nearly forgot to tell you about the – knickers. Not sure if I mentioned it before but in-flight for surgery purposes paper knickers always go under the gown. They always disappear after the operation – most disconcerting. On with flight 12 and under general anaesthetic Wingrave took my stent out. He then had me wheeled into the recovery room. I awoke to pain, blurred faces hovering over me and Wingrave bending down to tell me my ureter was in spasm.

More morphine got shunted in…. and again and again. Yes, my ureter had obstructed once more.

The porter wheeled me back to my room. Again he crashed into the bloody bedside table with the trolley.

More morphine got poured in.

I was rushed over to radiology.

More morphine.

Wingrave appeared, after radiology.

He told me I needed a 'perk' and then could go home. Having totally no idea what that meant I slept well and looked forward to breakfast and going home.

Next day, I was told I was 'nil by mouth'. Not even cup of tea more 'in flights gifts' of 'fresh' gown. Paper knickers too. For flight 13- short haul, same operating theatre, anaesthetic. This Doctor resembled a grumpy old fisherman in his sou'wester. He performed a nephrostomy.[7] Less morphine but tons of pethidine added to the mix.

In recovery I was vaguely aware that the catheter tap had not been closed. It leaked urine and blood everywhere. That caused one hell of a mess over the bed, floor, blanket, you name it. I was wheeled back by the same porter as the previous day. He hit the same bloody cabinet in the same bloody bed with the same juddering pain.

I was booked onto Flight 14 planned for the next week – long haul. But allowed home with a catheter bagged strapped to each leg. One from the kidney via the percutaneous[8] in my back and the other from my bladder via an indwelling catheter.

I found myself back in London for what I had begun to call my flights. Long-haul were the long operations. Short haul the short. Having been moved from Bedford hospitals, I found the London hospitals so much 'posher'. I likened the situation to comparing say economy (home hospital) with first (London hospital). I had been allowed

---

[7] A nephrostomy is a fine tube placed through your skin to drain a blocked kidney (Baus.org.uk).
[8] ibid.

home for the weekend and was now to get back to operations.

Flight 14 i.e., operation 14 took off on January 25th. Our ever-lovely taxi, Dick, took it upon himself to ask his wife to use his smart Mercedes and drive me from home to London. He thought that would be nicer for me to have a lady look after me. Such a brilliant driver was she, I even fell asleep, nephrostomy bag and all! Just as at Heathrow, we pulled up, she scuttled to the boot and as if by magic I floated from reception to my bed. Same old porter carefully carrying baggage and nothing too much trouble.

25 January 2011

The operation started late morning after a weird conversation Mr Wingrave. He seemed more worried about what to order for his lunch than anything else. I eventually arrived in the Critical Care Unit (CCU) at about 7:00pm. CCU was probably the most luxurious experience on offer anywhere in the world. Air bed, continual massage, every conceivable line, drain, tube and yes oxygen mask attached. Personal nurse on hand or toe! Every minute of every hour of every long day. Incredible experience. I spent 3 days in CCU then was moved into my own room on the ward where again, Comfy bed, TV, personalised menu, nursing, physiotherapy, fine dining and on and on. there were bumps and turbulence, few, unexpected infections, surprise allergies to antibiotics and other hurdles to overcome. As on a plane, however luxurious, whatever the class of travel, whatever the seat configuration, it is still, a plane. My wonderful airbed had a motor; in CCU it rumbled through my opiated brain, but once on the ward it took on the sound of a reverse thrust engine. I must have played my iPod 'all songs' A to Z every night as I attempted to drown out the noise of my bed!

Knickers. As before this became a bit of an issue! I was issued with those in-flight paper knickers which mysteriously disappeared after the operation. In a desperate bid for independence, I texted husband D. I asked him to bring some old baggy pants for me. These he dutifully found, six pairs in fact and popped them into a Tesco bag before leaping onto the next train. He arrived at the hospital sadly, NO knickers. He must have left them, all six of them, on the train. What a panic of embarrassment. We had visions of a bomb squad blowing up a suspect package! Evening Standard headlines: 'Knick Knickers Knicked'.

Caring for me was a brilliant nurse, the most amazingly funny night nurse who found a way to distract me from the panic of my anaphylactic reaction to a type of antibiotic. Then there was another nurse, who hid me from the crazy 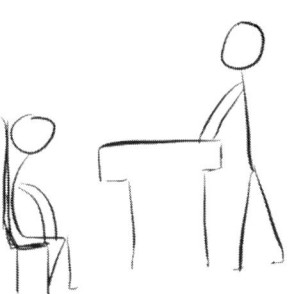 physios by wheeling me into the bathroom attached to all the drips, tubes and drains!

And the question was…now what? Well, my shark-attack-type-scar, drain tap on my back and bag strapped to my leg testified to the fact that this had been a complicated operation. I now had a newly re-implanted ureter in my bladder. My right kidney was however, dilated. I had to be booked onto another operation, number 15 on 8th Feb to insert two more stents.[9] Short haul flight 15 saw the introduction of a double stent to replace the single stent of January's massive operation. Wingrave had organised his colleague to sort the stents. For the purposes of this story his name is Jerome. Having never met me, nor I him, this extraordinary, lovely man rang me at home. 'I have never operated on someone I had not met before' he started the conversation. we chatted. Reassured I slept brilliantly before setting off to meet this kind empathetic surgeon. I arrived as instructed at his hospital at 5.00 am, a Club World sort of experience, at its best 'the flexibility to sleep, work or relax so you arrive refreshed and ready for the day / night ahead featuring the world's fully flat bed?!

---

[9] Stent: A ureteric stent is a thin, flexible tube which is curled at both ends to avoid damaging the kidney and urinary bladder and to prevent it from dislocating. The stent is placed so that its upper end is in the kidney and its lower end is in the urinary bladder.

9 April 2011 ....

January and February disappeared in a fog of anaesthesia and painkillers.

By the end of March 2011 I had had yet another operation. Getting into the usual gown and evaporating paper knickers. wahey! The very lovely Jerome was going to extract the stents. My poor friends, family, neighbours and medical fraternity must be wondering how to unsubscribe from this saga. I was advised to go and check out the source of massive back pain., another London surgeon. This time a spinal surgeon. Another hospital. Another zillion radiation images. En route I rediscovered an old favourite bagel bakery and picked a few to take home.

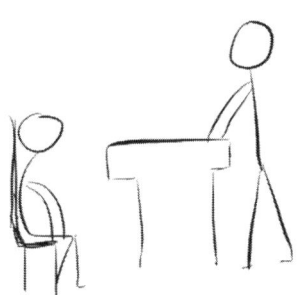

April 2011

Another admission form...the tiny space allowed for 'Please list any previous operations' made me giggle .... I left it blank!

Oh surprise? My spine had a tear, disc damage probably speeded up by 16 operations.

Wait for it.... Let's have general anaesthetic 17.... So that spinal surgeon can inject some amazingly brilliant substance into my back and with any luck that will work for 5/6 weeks he unsmiling told me. (He was not impressed with my admission form).

He smirked even more as he asked me to sign the consent form 'you'll be familiar with these' he chortled... In my haste to run/limp out onto the Finchley Road clutching bagels I had bought on my way in, and inwardly screaming my head off, I did not enquire as to what? Why? When? And then what?

December 2011

Well, well...I think I left you all wondering how the hell bagels and spines and kidneys ever got mixed up. Well, here's the story.... can you bear to read on? Short haul flights 17, 18 and 19 took place over May and June. These were 'minor' procedures to try to establish quite where the issues in the spine were. 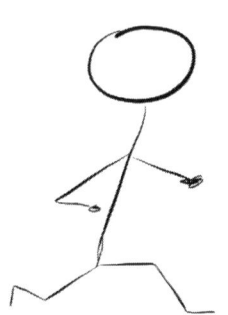 Each time I groggily rose from the anaesthetic I managed to imagine myself lying on a hot beach drinking cocktail. Never mind the oxygen mask, where was the snorkel when you needed it most? The hospital was really near an amazing bagel shop, which was such a treat.

February 2012

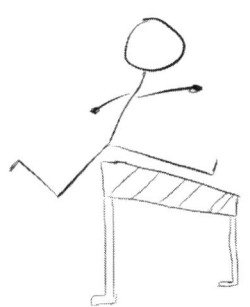 I think the last image you had from this blog was of a somewhat bedraggled figure clutching bagels down the Finchley Road. Well, my spinal

fusion[10] was in August 2011: pins, cage and bone graft firmly in place. I had to learn to walk again. Hours and hours of physio. It seemed ok. As it turned out unfortunately my bladder was apparently now 'denervated'—that meant it had lost all feeling. There was a massive problem. Having managed a brilliant reconstruction of my ureter to bladder but my ureter had no non-return valve as such…. As the bladder filled the urine went up to kidney and back down again in a rather glorious yoyo action. All the while, this was building up a great infection filled bladder soup. Antibiotics and painkillers were scaling new heights and less and less effective. Hospital admissions, instillations of drugs and actually it had all been a bit rubbish.

I had however put in a few teaching hours – a great distraction with endlessly patient colleagues ever at hand to lift, fetch, carry, supply hot Danish pastries and copious coffees. Fantastically pragmatic students: Who would do anything as long as the bribe was chocolate.

February 2012, a leap year, began with the suggestion from London that I should consider my options. With continued pain, infection, sepsis risk and a kidney in reflux most of the time. Five options emerged. Best one was 'do nothing'. Grounded! I really hoped we could take that one. Others involved moving all the right side to the left side in various guises. That sounded horribly lopsided to me, and I really could not contemplate any more major surgery. It sounded dramatic but actually it

---

[10] Spinal fusion is a major surgery and medical procedure used to treat back injuries. The surgery includes using rods and screws, and bone grafts to stabilize the spine.

was the least bad option. It was the least invasive, it was the least time in hospital. Least problematic recovery. I was to have the right kidney removed. Kidney Surgeon Prof Nick was amazing. He had grilled me on my intentions. He had checked my resolve. Ultimately, I was set for take-off again. Someone somewhere out there, was packing a bag ready for a new kidney and new beginnings – I wished them every happiness and best of health. It was a good kidney and just needed a ureter really. Maybe one day, I hoped, we might be allowed to share our stories. The operation took place on 29th Feb 2012. A date forever etched in my mind. The retrieval team assured me they would taxi the kidney across London. I have no idea why I was so adamant they did not go on the tube! The recovery was not too bad. Six weeks. The magic 6! Both Prof Kidney and Wingrave, assured me I had made the right decision. Jerome had also helped me come to the decision by writing a long email explaining the pros and cons and offering to speak to the various surgeons. On the day of the operation, he wrote again simply to wish me well and to thank me for giving the gift of life to a stranger. I just burst into tears.

Spinal November 2012 Flight Number 18

Spinal Stabilisation. Unexpectedly I found myself back in hospital, the discs at L4/5 were fused but L3............4 was bulging badly. I really thought I was in for just a quick procedure, but it ended up more difficult and a stabilisation was fitted at L3 and L4.[11] I had to get the black spinal corset on again and drugged up to the eyeballs relearn how to walk, bad leg down stairs and good leg leads to heaven bad to hell. The leading leg training for all back surgery.

February 2013

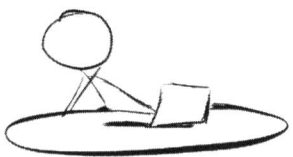

I now had to self-catheterise 4 hourly. As we all know catheters in-dwelling were invented 300 years ago and go hand in hand with horrible UTI's with increasingly resistant bug (ger) s treated with increasingly nuking puking antibiotics. Jerome, assured me research and development into the catheter thing was underfunded but ongoing – oh, yes? Catheters just are not the groovy charity inspirational thing, are they? One day I'm going to change that. My earth-shattering discovery from Jerome was that a 'domestos' wash-out via catheter to bladder of the hospital grade antibiotic 'Gentamicin'[12] for an hour a week, would possibly kill the bugs, no side effects, avoids oral antibiotics, is cheap, easily administered (via self-same catheter) and oh …. It worked well. So far so good. I shared this news with my friend Mel Reid who writes for the Times and every Saturday her column called Spinal Column. Her writing covers all the issues

---

[11] The vertebrae of the lumbar spine are labelled, L 1 L2 L3 L4 and L5.
[12] intravesical gentamicin instillations – introducing hospital grade antibiotics known as gentamicin directly into the bladder via catheter.

she and other spinal injury patients endure. She supports me in so many ways, writing to me, chatting, laughing. She too knows catheters only too well!

Blog entry May 2013

You.will.not.believe.it or maybe you will. …. My gallbladder was threatening to erupt. I can hardly bear to tell you May 10th at yet another hospital I was booked for a gall bladder op. This I promised myself, would be the LAST EVER operation…. Ready for take-off again.

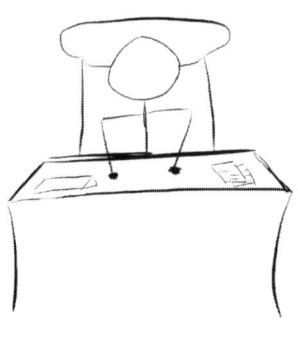

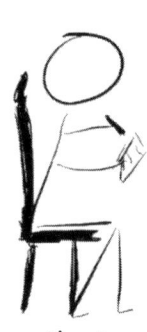

On the advice of the fantastic Jerome … and Montmorency…., I have been seen in the Allergy clinic on a few occasions. Facing a variety of skin tests and then challenging tests of potentially reactive substances which are thought to be reactive is as stressful as any of the horrendous operations I have had. Other patients must be more ill than I am and must face even worse fears. By explaining the dosage, the rationale, the evidence base and the outcomes the team include patients in decision making and 'ownership'. I faced the consequence of being allergic to increasingly few available anit-biotics capable of beating my recurrent infections. To be reassured and included in the process of elimination, crediting the patient with a degree of intelligence, adds value and confidence in the outcomes. Some consultants (none of those mentioned here) in my care, can be dismissive, somewhat cavalier in their explanations. That is not helpful and only diminishes confidence. The Allergy Team has made the situation so much better, and have explained their rationale, their solutions. Above all else they give the impression that they genuinely care about each and every patient. They seem to want to know the outcomes and go out of their way to keep in touch. In the busy life of a hospital doctor, I really do not know how they manage. But manage they do, even remembering from appointment to appointment the smallest detail. When the clinic is overcrowded, shared with another unrelated medical team and with no bays or beds, the little things really matter. The offer of a cup of coffee being one tiny example. The addition of a great deal of humour, is a considerable bonus! I wrote to the CEO: *cannot say enough to you, to urge you to pour every and any resource into this clinic and recognise the extraordinary team that is providing an extraordinary service to the benefit of patients and ultimately the NHS every time.*

BUDGET NHS Air. An email from Jerome to me
Tue, 18 Nov 2014

Letter from Jerome:

BUDGET-NHS-AIR There is always some food (often soup) on the table in every patient's room whenever I visit a patient. I thought they served it half-hourly rather than at random so that is another interesting observation / insight. At least you have been flying first class with BA. Imagine what it is like when folk fly

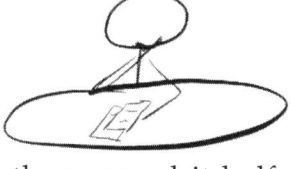

BUDGET-NHS-Air. They get a cup of warm water, left too far from the bed to reach. Of course, it is free at the point of delivery, but the plane is hopelessly overbooked, only staffed by one pilot and a trainee cabin crew, and subject to frequent cancellations. Turbulent air flow within the passenger cabin is a substantial hazard. Their plane has only got one wheel, one wing, and half an engine. Of course, it does not fly straight. This is something the government has investigated and, in fact, is not true. All BUDGET-NHS-Air jets have two or more wings, four or more engines, and are fully staffed with 3 pilots and eighteen cabin nurses per client. A new flight overseeing management infrastructure is being instituted to provide compulsory direction, training and most importantly motivation to the lazy pilot and trainee cabin crew member to fly the plane more efficiently and effectively. They have been told to audit their own performance and feedback to themselves, and devise their own, new, innovative ways of working. BUDGET-NHS-Air management will take appropriate credit when the time comes for their managerial prowess. Sadly, owing to procurement regulations, and new budget arrangements, the new two-winged, multi-engine aircraft have not yet been commissioned from the newly established primary air trusts. These will be delivered as part of the 2020 upgrade. In the meanwhile, the pilot can simply work harder.

Get well soon!

Letter to hospital Tue, 18 Nov 2014

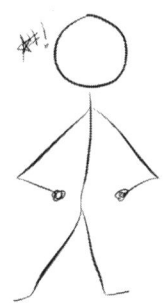

Dear Mr, I am writing to try to understand an unfortunate night at your hospital this week. I was admitted on Monday 7 July 2014, for a CT myelogram. In view of my allergies a protocol had been established with the help of your allergy team. Consultant Radiologist as in charge of the procedure and the allergy protocol. The team came up to my room and explained everything sympathetically and clearly. As you can imagine my previous experiences with contrast dye reactions have made me anxious about the whole thing. It has taken a great deal of persuasion and planning to organise the CT. The CT was done in the morning. I appreciate the huge amount of planning and time taken over this, along with all the various personnel who were in radiology for the event. Thank you very much. Everybody was fantastic. Back on the ward I was looked after by my appointed nurse. She was brilliant. She organised strong pain relief (oramorph) for my spinal pain, she checked for allergic reaction regularly and did frequent observations keeping a close eye on the situation. By about 8 pm I was becoming very hot and unwell. She called the Outreach team and very quickly it was decided in view of the allergic reaction further antihistamine should be administered IV. They were calm and solicitous to both myself and my poor anxious family who have seen it all happen before. Things became more stable and able to leave for the day. The night nurses then took over. Clearly, they were tired, stressed, and unhappy. For some reason they decided I could not have any oramorph. One of them, I am sorry I do not know her name, could not get my blood pressure reading. After several attempts with alarm bells jangling from the equipment, she started telling the machine to 'shut up'. Eventually she realised that she needed to plug the cuff into the leads to make it work. At about 11.00 pm. One nurse told me I did not need a catheter, in fact I must self-catheterise using CISC regime using disposable catheters, details of which must be in my records. Morning arrived and with it the day staff. What a contrast to the night staff. He immediately helped me feel reassured, calmer and less vulnerable. He was sympathetic, solicitous, and making checks on my allergies all the time. He found ways to make the itching better and rebuilt my confidence. Whilst in hospital, I really did not want to make a fuss and complain about fear of reprisals. Now that I am home and feeling so much better just writing the letter helps sort out the story in my own mind. During the night I did not feel safe in hospital. I do not know what else was going on for the staff. They clearly were having a difficult day and their stress transference made my vulnerability all the worse. They were agitated and perhaps needed some help themselves. I am quite sure they are normally fine and certainly my experiences of nursing at the hospital have never been like this before. Thank goodness for the day staff whose confidence, calm and safety made for a quicker recovery? I am not sure what you can do about this. I just think those poor nurses need some help and really should not be working in their agitated state. I would hate for other patients to suffer the same way. Yours sincerely

2014 Well here we were again back in medical land. After 5 years of this I was now eligible for NHS Pain Psychologist. This was suggested by the Pain Clinic who offered me a basket of help… acupuncture, anaesthetic patches, and psychology, drop-in advice clinic…. I readily agreed to everything.

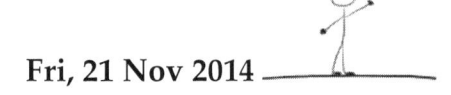

Fri, 21 Nov 2014

I went to my first psychology appointment. I was cynical and grumpy about psychobabble stuff… in my mind I was thinking stereotypical lies on the couch and muttering meaningfully. How wrong could I be? Dr Psycho turned out to be the sort of person I would count amongst my friends happy to chatter away about absolutely anything and everything. She indeed offered a couch or floor, or cushion should pain be too bad. The relaxation tape she gave me is so good I never have got past the first 3 seconds. The idea of pacing turns out to be to walk for 5 minutes then rest. Then next week 5 1/2 minutes then rest. You know? I really cannot do that. So, she says for the bonkers patients, like me, we would try to log a typical couple of days and work out which bits cause most pain which bits I really could leave till another day. OK I would try I needed to make time. Oh well…she is utterly lovely, says that some people arrive and need to be coaxed into talking. No problem there.

She says one lady was so good at mastering the coping strategies. She did not go out with her friends one night because she had not done the relaxation tape. Mm I think I have some way to go on this one. Still, it is a very jolly hour in great company with much laughter.

I'LL TOSS HIM A BONE Fri, 21 Nov 2014

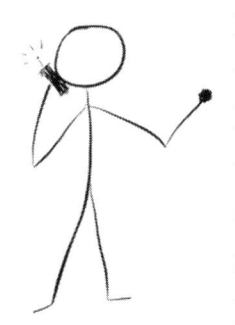

Now medical-wise things were a bit tricky. Having had a difficult summer in Milton Keynes hospital. Ha. Not me but this time my mother. made me realise some of my new-found skills on the medical front. There I was suggesting pain relieving remedies, requesting fluids, mouth wash and designing my own home made drugs chart for her. In the nicest possible way but so determinedly, to make things better. As for me, back pain and UTIs just would not shift. The ever-amazing Jerome had made great efforts to find other consultants to help and, in the meantime, had taken to distraction therapy. He said he could not cure me. (Tsk) but he could make me laugh. So, in a letter to all sorts of doctors and nurses all whose names begin with J, he signed off…That it looked like 'Three men in a boat'. He made the comment that henceforth he would be known as Jerome, remembering the author of said book and 'not forgetting the dog'. The distraction therapy continued by text with various references to the story, to the 'shirt in the river'. He even decided that our shaggy dog-like microbiologist could be Montmorency. As for Montmorency's involvement, 'Jerome' says: I will toss him a bone. From planes to boats…!

I continued my very part time teaching sixth formers on Tuesday and Home School children on a Friday. I was pretending to be a teacher with no pain, no issues, just an ordinary busy old school person. My blog entry stated: *I think I am still the person I was. But I crawl home, pop some pills, lie on the floor, and remember who I am now.*

During 2014 I underwent various tests including urodynamics.[13] Urodynamics is the most undignified of tests I know. The action takes place in radiology. A catheter goes into the bladder. A sensor goes into the bowel. The bladder is filled with saline (water) and the patient is encouraged to cough and pee standing sitting lying down with the clinicians watching. It is dreadful. It did however prove what I already knew that I could not empty my bladder fully if at all. I was taught how to self-catheterise in a brief lesson in the hospital. Grabbed my sample pack and went home to try on my own. So difficult to do at the start. In the hospital I had been taught to do it lying down. Who the hell pees into a toilet lying down? Standing or sitting i.e., the normal pose and finding the right place to get the catheter in. After a while I did it and never looked back.

By December 2014 I Had begun to be involved in public speaking. Patients rarely agree to talk about bladders. This one of the last taboos. I was persuaded to attend a parliamentary dinner at Westminster.

---

[13] Urodynamics tests are designed to show how your bladder is or is not working. See: https://www.baus.org.uk/_userfiles/pages/files/Patients/Leaflets/Urodynamics.pdf.

Nervous and worried that I would have nothing to say I travelled by train reading and rewriting my speech. My newfound friend with many connections in the world of Bladder Health had put my name forward. We were to go together. But in the event, I went on my own as she had just accepted a position with a supplier of catheters. A potential conflict of interest. I texted her all the way. What would I say? I have no idea what they want to hear? Just tell your story she replied.

Blog entry Wednesday 10th December 2014

I found myself seated at a Parliamentary Dinner at the House of Commons. The discussions were tightly steered by an excellent chair. Those present included MPs, surgeons, NHS England Chief Nurse, NHS England representatives, patient advocates, British Association of Urology Nurses, Consultant Urologists to name but a few. I started my story by talking about BC and AC …Life Before Catheters (BC) and Life After Catheters (AC). I managed my bladder and numerous UTIs that went hand in hand with my condition mostly well. Life was not simple. Even short trips had to be meticulously planned. I gave a short explanation of life since the 2009 hysterectomy. I included the day I was told I would have to self-catheterise. I explained my new bladder implant…a Sacral Nerve Stimulator (SNS). I told them I had been able to nurse my mother through cancer this year. She was more worried about having a catheter than losing her breast. I told them this was a taboo that needed to be broken. I reflected that cancer can be spoken about but continence not. I made them laugh by saying that as a child I did not think my mother knew the word breasts. But now, thanks to awareness campaigns we could say BREAST loud and clear. But what about BLADDER or BOWEL?

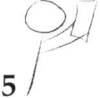

NEW YEAR resolutionsSat, 24 Jan 2015

Here we were another New Year, another raft of resolutions.

> Resolution
> 1: avoid surgeons – already failed
> 2: get fitter – swim spin…
> 3: less unpaid work – negotiating.
> 4: Ski. aha well, good start. Did something horrible to my back and ended up with an emergency scan 23rd Dec… The 'Mr Hypodermic' insisted I see old Boring Ben the spinal surgeon. So, I had to see him he as chatty (not) as ever. In his opinion the disc

At L2/3 was bulging and so he reasoned, all our worrying that should he have extended the fusion maybe was right. Nuclear scan next, as MRI is impossible due to SNS. Lovely letter from the esteemed Jerome. Thanking me for the Three Men in a Boat book I had sent him at Christmas.

Urodynamic tests had again been scheduled. This time next at a new (to me) hospital… Good for the bagel shop and spectacularly nice kind understanding team. Dipstick, the new surgeon in the boat was in attendance. He had insisted on allergy protocol and overnight stay. The test itself is gruesome and as before the oft repeated 'Tell us when you feel 'full' as in bladder just does not happen. Upside down, turned all around, stand, sit, whirl…still nothing…difficult to. Cough. Leak. Reflux. Mm.

In 2015, I began to accept invitations to speak at continence events. These are usually sponsored by a supplier and patient stories, I am told, are invaluable to the assembled clinicians.

Mastermind. February 2015

Another month of continuous UTIs and antibiotics that made me feel like slitting my throat which was marginally better than the horrendous spasms that made me feel like slitting my bladder. A cunning plan evolved master-minded by the legend that is Jerome. The idea was to be admitted to hospital, get some IV antibiotics in, and try to break this endless cycle of infections. The duty doctor who clerked me at admission, announced somewhat conspiratorially that he thought I had an infection. No? Really? Sherlock. He further suggested a course of wait for it… Antibiotics … And I was discharged home. Jerome answered my perplexed and tearful texts and calls … Here is his summary of events….

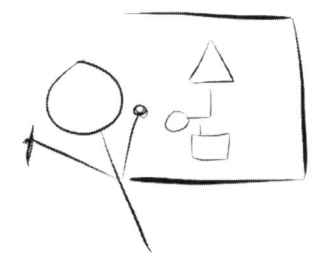

'Dear all

Some thoughts regarding our mutual patient JE. The plan for admission for inpatient assessment and treatment – including a bit of respite from the burdens of managing an almost continuously symptomatic UTI for months, despite equally continuous oral antibiotics was, I think, a good idea. – As you know and have discussed together already, this was scuppered by the somewhat premature discharge back home today with the rather familiar plan of more oral antibiotics…. And a return trip from home back to London tomorrow. JE – as this is written in print it confirms that we are sorry that the plan was not executed more effectively So we need a clear strategy (and contingency) going forward as it is increasingly clear that oral antibiotics one after another have not improved, let alone solve, the problem Can we admit (as per original plan for yesterday) UNDER MY CARE for 72 hours in patient assessment. Book dates according to tests needed, in patient consultations needed, and, if agrees, IV ANTIBIOTICS JE has responded well to the prophylactic doses she has had IV when she has had procedures. Could there be an issue with oral absorption??? If IV abs worked, then maybe this could be an issue At least we (and especially JE) would know that she CAN be cleared of infections and symptoms.

bw

Jerome to the rescue. Awesome speed, empathy, efficiency, and humour. Aforementioned 'msu' hatched, matched, dispatched to aforementioned 'lab'. Then he told me about a dire morning briefing of his own. It was something like 'levity and brevity'. I had to ask him to repeat…. this is what he sent me:

*I liked the "hatched, matched and dispatched" for the MSU! My phrase was in response to a truly dour presentation I had to endure earlier that morning. Just as it had got into what is normally the middle part, it ended, almost mid-sentence, with just a blank slide…I texted a colleague to say: "At least, **what it lacked in levity it made up for with brevity**"….* bw

Sequin's 30 MARCH 2015 Sat, 04 Apr 2015
COMMISSIONING FOR QUALITY AND INNOVATION (CQUIN) NATIONAL GOALS.

NHS England Excellence in Continence Care (EICC)[14] Board. Here we were 6 years after this Odyssey in Uti- world started and I find myself sitting round the inaugural board table of the EICC programme. This was born of a chance encounter in the bowels (a deliberate use of the word) of the House of Commons. Chance? Well, an orchestrated lobby of MPs and NHS England by clinicians, patients, and producers My hastily written speech then, was based on the BC AC

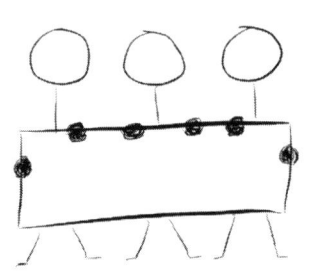

---

[14] https://www.england.nhs.uk/publication/excellence-in-continence-care/.

idea.... So, all I could think of to say was BEFORE Catheters and AFTER Catheters. To get the BC AC bit in for continence. The Lady Chair was efficient and good and restoring order. Children the country over must rest assured the passionate championing of their continence cause by specialist nurses was awesome. They were ferocious.... They were the bull terriers... Patients aged 18-70, hang on in there. We adult patients will do our level best. It could be so simple. Quality of products. Quantity. Assessment. Dignity. Self-referral/ control of own destiny.... they peered down their bespectacled noses at me. A patient? Speaking? I *must remember I am only a patient*. What on earth could I possibly know? My role as patient advocate at NHS England Excellence in Continence Care (EICC) began to take over my life! The only patient, I was co-opted to advise on new commissioning guidance, on behalf of all patients.

December 2015 was the launch of Excellence in Continence Care Guidance. () EICC). at the House of Commons. The All-Party Political Group (APPG) Continence were the hosts in a magnificent committee room. The outgoing chair of the Royal college of General Practitioners, Claire Gerada was there. A team from Public Health England. All of us from the EICC and MPs Lords and Ladies. As a result, I was invited to join the All-Party Parliamentary Group (APPG) for Continence[15] as a patient representative. Meetings have been held at Westminster House of Commons or House of Lords. I

---

[15] http://www.appgcontinence.org.uk/ All Party Parliamentary Group APPG for bladder and bowel continence care

pinch myself every time. What an amazing experience. wandering the corridors of power...talking about bladders. Who would have thought it? It is an honour and a privilege. I do not want that to sound trite. I mean it. I just hope I can somehow do justice to the faith placed in me.

GERMAN-DRUGS-BAN May-2015

Montmorency had discovered a new treatment successfully used in Spain. The evidence was anecdotal but that is the Spanish for you I was told. The product 'urovaxam'[16] was worth a try he said.

Email exchange Microbiologist to JE.

On 15 May 2015 16:26, Montmorency. Wrote to me.

Dear J (Re: Uro vaxom. I have worked on this issue. Should have been easy. Now turns out it is illegal to directly access. No pharmacy is now allowed to be an intermediary.in what is deemed an "unlicensed" medical product. HOWEVER, patients. Are allowed to purchase for their own needs. Working to find a target German pharmacy which can supply this; will pass this info on to you together with a script for the vax. You then e mail them with my script, they will ask you for a credit card number (should not cost too much) and then they will send directly to you.... (Please stand by Thanks.

---

[16] https://www.uhs.nhs.uk/AboutTheTrust/Newsandpublications/Latestnews/2020/February/Researchers-say-vaccines-could-substantially-reduce-recurrent-urine-infections.aspx.

Jerome replied: Illegal indeed. Wow. It seems like possessing vs distributing cannabis… (You could have made M into a common criminal simply through his trying to help. Goodness knows how long it would take to identify a suitable German pharmacy if he is doing time at her majesty's displeasure… (Bonkers. You need to tell NHS England about this. If you get the stuff and use it, under the direction of a doctor (it was not your idea after all) what difference does it make if you pay on credit and get it direct or turn up at your local pharmacy and hand them a bundle of used notes. They should sort this out. It is ridiculous. Meanwhile, as I come down from rant city, I hope you are feeling a bit better. (I have got your file and will send some MSU forms for you to put with a sample as and when you need to use them. I Hope to go out next week. Have a better weekend than last. Best wishes Jerome.

LOST Blog entry 18-May-2015

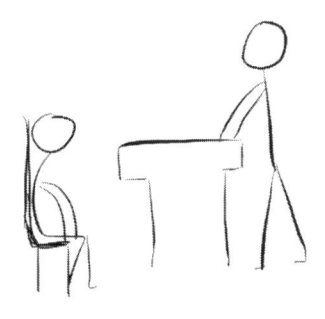

The Neuromodulator[17] team assessment with psychologist and clinical nurse specialist was today. It seemed I had got 'lost' in their system, hence long delay. Oh well. Typical scenario. I had sent an email to the Consultant in charge-

---

[17] A spinal stimulator delivers mild electrical pulses to the nerves to interrupt the transmission of pain signals to the brain, thus reducing pain. https://northernpaincentre.com.au/wp-content/uploads/2020/06/8195_Patient_QAs_1662020.pdf.

with a copy of my last urology letter. The 'system.' had lost the record of my consultation with It cannot proceed without assessment and group workshops which are every Monday for four weeks. I am now on that list for September. Neuromodulator sometime after that. That was good because if I opted for urology intervention that would be best first, they said. They also mentioned how great it would be for urology and pain clinics to communicate on this. As if they ever would! It was gruelling but the Consultant was great. The Specialist nurse though, kept firing questions at me. *Why didn't I take higher doses of painkillers? Why did I have a boari flap operation twice or a 'flap'* as she called it peering down her spectacles –? I felt defensive and ended up doubting my desired aim to reduce not increase painkillers. As for the boari flap etc. it is not as if I woke up one morning and thought' I know' I'll ask a surgeon to chop me and my bladder up today… 'She challenged my use of diazepam, which had been advised by the Pain team at Milton Keynes. And indeed, the Consultant Pain and his team. That is, it was not me randomly trying to class A drug. She also queried why I thought the drugs made me so dopey. She said I could be on much higher levels. I do not want to be an 'at home zombie'. That is why I'm doing this. I worked hard to get to this level of drugs. I had endured migraine crazy days of too-much-too fast gabapentin.[18] *Was I sensitive*? She asked. Well trying not to sound rude I was not before but now I am. I think she

---

[18] a pain killer gabapentin is used for nerve pain and has side effects of dizziness, fatigue and tired.

meant drugs! Full of renewed self-doubt. Was this all my fault after all? The brilliant Psycho Sue had got me out of that mind set. Then it was the turn of the Mr Hypodermic's Psychologist, who was gentler than the interroga-interrogation nurse. How old are my four children? That is a question I try to avoid and feign vagueness. Not happy with that, she wanted exact ages. The eldest two are the same age does not mean they are twins. I had to explain all that again. Yes, we brought up our HIV / AIDS orphaned NEPHEW. We have encountered dying many times. Yes, our nephew calls us Mum and Dad and we are fiercely protective of him and very proud of ALL four. No, that does not make me an emotional wreck. He makes me feel lucky. Teaching cropped up when the children were older … we are a family know we can meet disasters and survive and even laugh again. We can do this…

The nurse interrupted yet again…She queried my use of the local anaesthetic plasters…recommended by Dr Pain man at MK. ….and so it went on… The interrogation began at 1:00 ended at 3:15 missed train home… Argh. But maybe they played a 'good cop bad cop' to test patient resolve to opt for Neuromodulator and not drugs or operations?

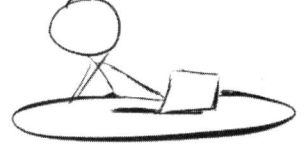

Hope all is well. Thank you for all your support…

Jerome-replied 20.5.15.

Jerome wrote:

Wow. What so many clinicians forget is that there are real life people, with real life lives, behind all our consultations. Consultations impact far more deeply, wider, and for longer than they do on the clinician ("next please") …. But even this level of understanding looks like genius compared with the trite soundbites of the politicians. An NHS with time to care. What a crock of shite. It takes hours and hours with a patient (as we have) to get to see and hear insights like yours. I could never have this with everyone – it is just not doable. It has been built over years of communications and understanding. It transcends the normal doctor patient interaction but gives so much insight into what it is like to be on the receiving end of treatments especially surgery. Thank goodness you are representing the patient on the NHS England board. You were advised to have a Boari flap. That is all there is to it – following the prior operation that did not go so well…

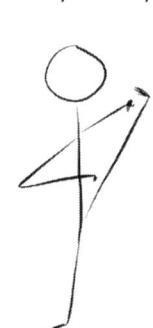

Meanwhile, but not meant in any sort of mitigation / defence or even an explanation of your predicament, consider the extraordinary job that it is to be a surgeon. What an unbelievable responsibility to make a decision, take the unswerving trust and faith of another person, and operate on them. in the hope that things will be better, but knowing that in an unfortunate few, they may not or get worse… How, when we understand the deeper consequences of our failures to help, can we ever pick up tools and do the same for another patient seeking our advice. It is not like medicine where we can say this pill did not work; let us try

another one. We know it is our own work that has let the patient down. We are told to reflect and have appraisal, but, as you say, there are evil people out there pretending to be nurses or doctors, or even real ones that prey on children, who do not get weeded out by these laborious processes until it is already way too late. The system. Is crazy. The people who care, care too much, and could not cope with knowing too much about the negative implications of some of their decisions, actions, or omissions. The problem, with a politically run NHS is it does not have the guts to admit that it simply cannot live up to its promises. And it just keeps making more and more. The patient is not like a car going in for a service (why did you get the carburettor changed; you needed a new exhaust) ... You cannot simply get a new one if the engine is too difficult to fix. The system is slow, too complicated, lies about being patient centred (3 days' notice – nice – who books a holiday with 3 days' notice? Or a show? Or even a dinner out with friends?) And asks too much of both the staff and, more importantly, the patient. It needs both to fight to get things done. Both are ready for the challenge in a proper doctor patient partnership, but neither needs the false promise that it is easy, quick, and certainly not guaranteed. Or some nurse you have never met asking you to justify someone else's decision that can't be changed anyway. It all sounds rather horrendous to me…I will send 10 MSU forms and keep my bit as simple, reliable, and helpful as I possibly can. In the meanwhile, I hope you have a decent sleep as a better remedy even than neuro modulation courses and will look out for replies at 0600 or thereabouts as we both tackle the next day at the front line of healthcare (provider and seeker and real-life receiver).bw Jerome

The Men in the boat meet up. Blog entry 25 June 2015

I rushed off to a joint meeting of all the surgeons in the boat. I don't recall being so worried so dry mouthed before a consultation. And I have had a few! Surgeons including Dipstick and Jerome vs Daniel Me.

They were good, better than good, brilliant. We talked about taking the bladder out of the equation. Literally. Conduits and stomas.[19] Weirdly my newfound knowledge from conferences meant I knew what that meant. Goodness knows what poor D thought. We considered risks. We thought about doing nothing. Doing nothing meant continuous UTI issues. Ever increasing resistance to antibiotics, threat of sepsis, spinal disc degeneration as previously and higher pain medication. A spinal fusion on the horizon if we did not get that under control. As ever various risks. As ever the only one you, the patient and he, the patient's husband, hear is: 'mortality'. There is no nice way of putting it. But as I said later that night. I think there is a higher mortality rate driving down the M1. So, with surgeons rushing off to save more lives we were left with Dipstick to summarise by Dictaphone, his letter. A very good way to include patients in the process of understanding. I found his attempts at humour disconcerting, he commented that I clearly had a good relationship with my husband and could sit on a professional body. What on earth has that got to do with it? Should I be satisfied with that? Should I just sit at home doing voluntary service and

---

[19] A stoma is created in the abdomen to allow the ureter to carry urine from the kidney into a stoma bag outside the body.

caring for my husband? I am not sure what he was referring to. He also asked if we were insured. Our response did not seem to meet his required response. Yes, we are insured. But he said the insurer would be unlikely to pay him the required fee. He would expect us to pay £5000 or so ourselves. I have never heard a surgeon go for the money side like that before. Yes, Daniel said, we will pay if we have to. Two surgeons, two fees? We could go to the NHS, but he said his appointments are booked out beyond the next year. His operating lists are running 18 months from referral. That was not a choice then. Was it?

24 hours continued MAY 2015

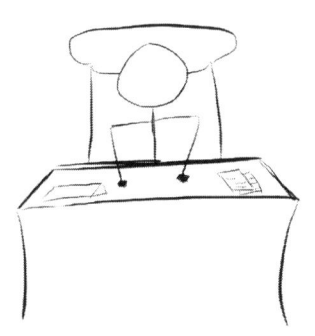

One minute I was coordinating a team of secondary teachers needing programming skills for a new curriculum, next I was in Battersea in a smart hotel. Guest of a supplier I had a sumptuous room slept like a log feeling better than I had for a few weeks now. Guest speaker for urology live event. Nurses' physios from hospitals across Southeast. My speech much like others I have done and documented previously was 'my story' but suffice to say I cannot make it sad or serious. Is that called denial? Everyone with a bladder and bowel problem should be listened to and should have access to the right care, treatment and support to make my goal a reality, people with a bladder and bowel problem must be offered high quality information about their condition and treatment and care. Be fully involved in the decision about their treatment and care and be treated with dignity and respect. Have access to interventions that have been recommended by national guidance. Be offered a full assessment by an appropriately trained professional and a personalised care plan which is reviewed at regular intervals.

I mentioned my swimming too. I started last year when my youngest, BFG was recovering from injury to his knee and me with spine injury. My running days are over. So, as I told the conference delegates open water swimming is highly recommended. My wet suit was so tight it was a workout in itself to squeeze on. Then the compression effect holds all the painful legs back and pelvis in one place. The water was so damned cold a sort of ice bath anaesthetic. Oh and no worries about that leaky bladder. In fact, any leaks were quite warming and out in the open. It was wonderfully, relaxing and just so addictive. My final words to the audience: I am honoured to be here today. And grateful for the opportunity to raise awareness about a subject that has certainly changed my life. Although I am bewildered to find myself here at all…I still do not quite believe it myself……

Blog entry: Update from House of Commons Sun, 19 Jul 2015

Thursday saw the launch of a Better Bladder campaign called 'Its Personal' at the House of Commons. The campaign brought together charities and patients The goal of this campaign was simple: everyone.

> with a bladder and bowel problem should be listened to and should have access to the right. care, treatment and support for them.

But first to share with you terribly sad news that at the start of week Di my friend and maths colleague was in a fatal car crash last Sunday. It was unbelievably sad. Hit hard. The last conversation we had had. Ironically, we had laughed at the name of a consultant she was seeing at a nearby hospital. So inappropriate I cannot possibly divulge. We shared self-catheterisation jokes. Botox for bladder induced much hilarity. As she was going for it and hoped for a face bot too! I'd told her about the personal launch. She'd have loved it… House of Commons? Nah. She'd have been in the Lords as Lady Di. Dammit. So, Thursday with mixed emotions and a crashing headache off to Westminster I went …. the full story will follow.

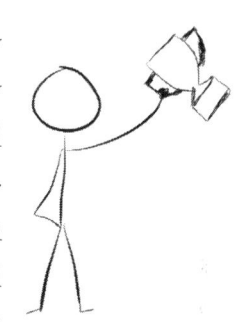

Westminster Tue, 04 Aug 2015

We needed to get 20 MPs to sign up to get the bill relating to Continence Care for November Parliamentary debate. Great news was that Melanie Reid Times columnist who had been in touch via a mutual friend had kindly agreed to support the campaign. That was great because a) she is awesome and very much a catheter user. b) She has a media presence c) she is humble and d) grounded in common sense.

NHS England is gearing up for a meeting with the Director of Children's services to tell him to stop CCGs from removing paediatric community continence services. My brain buzzed with ideas how we could make this better.

Pay up Wed, 05 Aug 2015

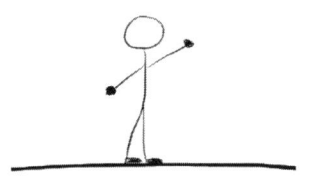

An email had arrived from surgeon Dipstick He was refusing to go ahead with the big operation until and unless I organised guaranteed funding for an intensive care bed after the operation. He had in fact cancelled the operation i.e., he had thrown his toys out of the pram, again. Could I sort it? .... oh shhhhhhh. After many phone calls and careful explanations. I fixed it with the insurers. We were covered. The operation was back on.

Blog entry: Just a little scratch. Tuesday 11th August 2015

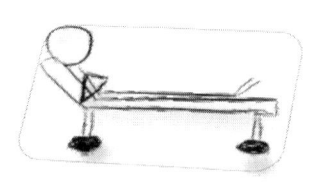

Up early then scurried round at home. Freezer filled? Check. Washing and ironing done? Check. Bins out? Check. Neighbours help note, patio watered blah. CHECK. Before I knew it, the taxi had whisked me to the train station. It could almost have been to get to Luton airport for a flight to...? My baggage on board along with all the other holiday makers. Only thing was, they got off at Luton Airport and I sailed on to glorious St Pancras. My favourite station. Carefully ignoring the wonderful coffee smells, on account of the nil by mouth, preoperation instructions, I made my way through the Grand Hotel reception and allowed the porter to signal up a cab. Have a nice flight he said as he waved me off. I arrived at the hospital, and I made my way through check-in, passport control, and security Nurse completed the boarding procedure. Surgeon 1 Wingrave, visited with kind sympathetic noises. Just right. Consent form rapidly completed. Goodness knows what I signed up for. He said Surgeon 2 aka Dipstick, would typically not turn up til the last minute and would moan about Wingrave. He also added that Dipstick usually took ages to operate but he, Wingrave, operated speedily. Which would I rather I pondered? Help... He wandered off to start his 'list'. RMO arrived with general assessment ECG etc. Phlebotomist arrived next. Blood sample taken for the click and collect. 'Just a little scratch'. He was great. Actually, all phlebotomists are. Fabulous skill... Dipstick arrived! Moaned about Wingrave's economy of words on the consent form. Announced proudly that he cancelled the operation last week. Wondered whether I knew that? Looking weirdly at him I said yes indeed I did know as he had asked Jerome's secretary to email me with said news. No personal call no consideration of tense patient-counting-the-days-to-the-op. would it not have occurred to him that the patient might NEED to know it'd been cancelled? Anyhow after many phone calls playing the game of words on funding, I'd got it sorted and covered at the 11th stress hour. Off he went muttering about Wingrave. I guess as colleagues they could just moan about each other. Anaesthetist turned up. Wow. Nice empathic quick run through the flight plan, chatter about technology, preparing for imminent take off as the two surgeons were 'champing at the bit to get started'. Sure, enough seconds after he had left a nurse arrived, paper knickers. Check. Gown Check. Stockings Check. Nail varnish Check. My superstitious application of toenail varnish was missed. Contacts out Check. SNS turned off check. Go. Heart thumping, we walked the walk of fear to lift and into the vomit green painted anaesthetic room. Surrounded by 6 or so green covered aliens who fired questions at me. Allergies? Check. That took a while. Stumbled over my surname as ever. Fired more questions at me. Into sight loomed kindly anaesthetist. Winking whispering about iPads, he put cannula in easily, 'just a small scratch'. From somewhere behind me the two surgeons hovered, only eyes visible and appeared somewhere over my head. Cheerily patting my head?! And making encouraging noises. With another wink the anaesthetist showed me the magic big white filled syringe…. oblivion…hurrah… Next thing I remember? Excruciating pain everywhere. Mumbled noises all around … then oblivion once more. Next thing I was aware of was being on a trolley in a lift somehow attached to two sort of huge water filled balloons. The porter tripped as we came out of lift pulling the connecting tubes. I could not help but yell…agony descended once more. A Nurse rushed to my side twiddling with all the lines. Trolley was stopped once more... 'Your husband is in the relatives' room'. Into sight zoomed worried knackered looking D. Poor him. Two second hello and he was dispatched to the room of stress once more until I'm harnessed into the CCU unit. As I clutched my familiar pain reliever[20] button I pressed and pressed and pressed .... blessed oblivion descended again.

Day 1 WEDNESDAY 12

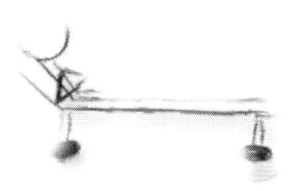

DAY 1 Wednesday 12th I was in CCU gradually waking up through the night. Such was my expertise, I recognised the unit having been the first patient in this new state of the art unit, some 4 years ago. At some point I must have been given my phone and had since learnt I sent a few gobbldy gook texts through the night. Goodness knows how. I do recall trying to read a message from D, just could not get my eyes to stay still long enough to read what I later saw was 'goodnight'. In a deja vu moment I sensed major preparations around me. The 6 a.m. bath. Goodness. How on earth the wonderful nurses do this I do not know. Dignity and empathy are adjectives that spring to mind, as they circumvent the many lines, wash off that orange surgery paint, changed sheets, gown and even remembered that essential, tooth brushing. At their

---

[20] Personal Analgesia Pump the patient can self-treat by pressing for pain relief

suggestion I had kept pressing the morphine pump to beckon oblivion once more. Surfacing at some point my legs felt like they'd been attacked by 100 mosquitos itching and itching. Nurse B hurried to my side. In seconds the magic potion is added to one of the lines and all calmed down. The day floated on. It was great. No one else was in the CCU. Nurses were there just for me. D popped in. Mr Surgeon 1 came…he explained the operation, all I could remember of that were the words tricky and oozing. With no idea what that meant I floated off once more. The CCU beds were a sort of air bed which the mattress pockets move, pocket by pocket ensuring constant massage effect. Legs encompassed in massaging boots which similarly keep squeezing the legs all the time on and off. D returned with some of the children. Their worried looking faces peering at all the jiggery pokery…I summoned some inner humour and talked about swimming in wet suits through the fog of morphine I heard them giggle and started a new story. Remembering not to hit the PCA* (personal controlled analgesia) so that I could stay awake …we laughed and chattered…at least I think I did….not forgetting that yet again those magical paper knickers had disappeared once more. It really is extraordinary. The food situation: Nil by mouth 2 cm water sipped over the day. More than that caused throwing up.

Blog entry Day 2 THURSDAY 13th

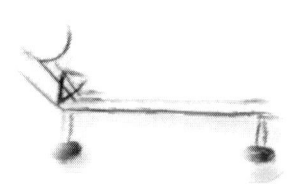

Dipstick came to see how I was doing. He too mentioned tricky op. He too mentioned oozing. I still did not know what he meant. Never mind. He also remembered to tell me that both of the surgeons, were away that weekend. They had organised a cover from their team. Clearer headed I cottoned on to the multifarious blood tests. My Daughter 2 came into CCU after work. She helped me with some communication that is she wrote some messages as my typing fingers seemed to have a mind of their own. She sent my dictated message to my brother in North America. Sometime previously Daniel and I had set up a comms system with my brother. We texted him. He then jollied up the message and ensured a positive spin. He would email a pre-listed group of close friends. He did not send e-mails to our panic-struck parents but spoke to them on the phone. This was a practice we adopted right at the start of all this in 2009. D found all the texts and phone calls too much to cope with, wouldn't we all? Daniel and George my youngest, arrived as a nurse came to tell me my haemoglobin had been dropping all day. Blood transfusions had been ordered. Did I consent to that? Don't know what any of that meant I just agreed. D kept telling his joke that I'm like athletes done for doping because they are getting more blood cells to make them. Run faster. I got confused. So, he told me again... I was also to be moved to the ward, with my very own two CCU nurses. How amazing was that? The hospital was closing CCU and all but one ward due to consultant holidays. So off we trooped…G and D worriedly trailed behind my rollerball bed and carried my only possessions – wash bag and drugs! D kept telling his joke that I'm like athletes done for doping because they are getting more blood cells to make them run faster……. Again, I was asked for transfusion consent…'It'll make you feel so much better'. I felt high as a kite and great actually. Better than what? What is the baseline? In any case I readily consented. Was I meant to check something before I did? Don't know. Is that just Jehovah's Witnesses? Even in my groggy state I was remembering that pre-op blood sample. 'Click and collect' I called it. Still cannot remember what that cross-matching thing is. Anyhow I did need it after all. Uh Oh. I had rotator massages on my legs. My bed was an air bed, which felt a bit like a waterbed. I had less tubes, not much has happened in my day. Surgeon 1, Wingrave, came in later. He had seen D and G leaving. Said he was surprised and confused at haemoglobin count. Oh well that made two of us. Said he was away for a week from now because of holiday. But had organised cover as Dipstick was also away until next week.

Food: nil by mouth. 2cm water only! Tasted like nectar. Really.

Day 3 and 4 Friday and Saturday

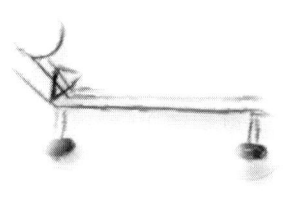

My friends from our 'Prosecco club' M and V, visited… Clearly, I'd been asleep on their arrival, and I juddered awake to their familiar voices whispering beside me. It was great to see them. I must have been asleep again as I woke later to find D and Daughter 2 had arrived with coffee (oh that tasted so good) especially as there was no sign of soup! Wingrave arrived and again said he would be away from now for a week or so. …

He told me he had appointed a Mr Bean, to cover.

Blood transfusions continued – 'that's a surprise, didn't expect that 'said Wingrave 'Mmm' said I

'That a good thing'

Was I feeling better? Wingrave asked.

'Don't know. 'Better than what?

DAY 4 Saturday 15th

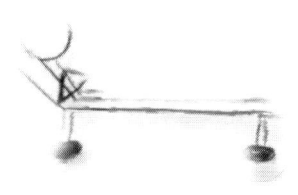

Surgeon Bean arrived, early morning. Introducing ourselves. Poor man 'whatamIdoinghere'. Nurse accompanied him. She smoothed things over and grinned at me…… Bean checked scars and dressings and beat a hasty retreat.

Breakfast. A grey kind of pungent slop and an icy looking sorbet or similar. Trying not to retch I boldly tucked in my napkin. One of the nurses came into my room, 'you not eating that whatever they be after doing?' to my relief she scooped it away.

BFG our name for George, visited. He made me laugh about lobsters and chickens…an old joke.

Then Miss Honey, my Cornish cousin, arrived bearing gifts…ginger jam, chilli sauce and a smoky scented candle.

The latter a nod to my pyrotechnic tendencies and the former an effort to cheer up the slop.

Evening brought true tomato soup 'diluted with water' the lady said. Tasted fine to me. TV on and Night Nurse T arrived. Spent ages working out the painkiller schedule and night routine. We made a great plan and called ourselves the 'A' team. She was brilliant. All night long.

Days 5 and 6 Sunday Monday

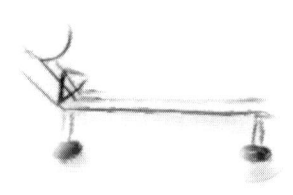

Sunday 16th Early morning. This was a bit more Deja vu: Mr Bean popped in early in the morning. Ducking all my questions he suggested I ask Wingrave and Dipstick to answer them when at least one of them returned…Poor man 'whatamIdoinghere'. … Checked scars and dressings then beat another hasty retreat.

'Eat anything you like' he added.

'Poor Mr Bean' I muttered 'suddenly you are in the boat of confusion'.

Breakfast: Natural yogurt. It was great. Progress was being made.

Not long after…you will not believe it the lovely nurses leapt over my bed like a flying gazelle…

'Surgeon's here' she muttered.

'Err, he's been' I confidently whispered.

The door flew open and who strode in …none other thanWingrave Himself. What Are They Like?

The conversation went something like this.

Hi. Hows you?

Great.

Great.

'Erm, we thought you were away' I managed to stutter out like an idiot.'

'No next week next week.

Right… Let's take out one of the catheters' he replied.

Oh? I mumbled Dipstick had said to leave two catheters in.

Mr Bean had agreed.

Help! I had understood I'd be going home with two. Argh. Help.

He joked, examined, checked scars and dressings then stayed bedside for a chat…

'Eat anything you like' he said.

Why on earth did they get poor Mr Bean to cover?

No sooner had he gone when like a sort of gurney, in trundled the catheter removal trolley, I recognised from many previous experiences.

I summoned up some inner courage and begged the nurses to ring Dipstick.

They did. He apparently agreed from afar that one catheter should indeed be removed. That went against all that he had told me. Conservative approach he had said. Time the great healer and all that. Dammit what was I meant to do?

J you-are-only-the-patient…I resigned myself to the inevitable… catheter was out although the suprapubic was left in.

Bogus. I hoped to goodness this was the correct decision. Help. What could I do? Frrrrrrr.

That afternoon somehow turned into a sort of party, well sort of! Miss Honey, AT, BFG, my Daughter 2, and their friends all turned up. I sat up, resplendent in my in bed. Visitors desperately tried to avoid eye contact with… catheter bag …. And … the drips and drains.

I was getting more mobile.

Walked from bed to bathroom. Whoop. What a feeling.

A Wonderful Ward Sister called Lizzie arrived. It had been noted that I had not eaten a lot. So, the catering manager. Yes… the CATERING MANAGER…. was sent to see me. Result.

It was understood I could eat.

'Eat anything you like' …well what would I like? she asked.

Don't know really. Soup? Toast? Be great.

Maybe some carroty chopped up veg kind of 'I said 'but really please don't worry. I am totally fine on coffee and watery tomato soup.

DAY 6 Monday 17th No surgeons visited today.

Phew. Jerome sent a message. He was just back from holiday. 6.30 am and he was messaging patients. Amazing. How the hell?

Anyway, my answer appeared to be something like:

'Hello J. Welcome back. Thank you. I'm not sure of the room or floor and currently harnessed to bed. I think it's 4ty something I'll confirm.

D and L arrived later. They were great company. Excellent visitors. Chatter. Reading. TV.

Other messages I managed to type out included. All going really well after' tricky' op. Men in boats cautiously optimistic. Opiate hallucinogenic making typing a sort of 3D experience…. nurses are fantastic, they think of everything even! Doing well here…they've taken down nearly every tube line and bags. Just going to have one catheter for a while until bladder reconstruction heals OK. It's fine, I really don't mind that.

Day 7 Tuesday 18th

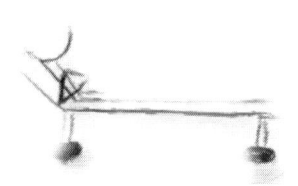

Dipstick turned up. Confirmed Wingrave had not been in touch. Agreed he planned to send me home with 2 catheters. But said it doesn't matter. Good that I asked the hospital to ring him over the weekend. Suggested I could go home Wednesday after stitches out. No need to check the scar etc. and depart. Seconds later the Registrar arrived. You have an infection he announced. Need antibiotics. Argh. Help I fumed. Just a minor hiccup surely. Pah. Don't tell anyone…just my brother thousands of miles away. He blamed a sudden onset of Tourette's for his response. That certainly matched mine. L popped in after work just down the road. She munched her healthy takeaway salad while I tried to order a small fudgy gift for nurses as a thank you. Eventually I got it.

I think morphine not only slowed me down it actually slowed down my laptop too which chose to freeze and lose my order n+1 times. Swapping jolly banter with L there was a knock at the door. Baffled nurses once more announced the arrival of yet another surgeon. Now who?

Hah. None other than awesome Jerome himself. Before he had even sat down there was a giggly story to repeat. No need to introduce him to L. Must be Mr x daughter guessed correctly. Well, no, just call me Jerome he instructed. Well, we chattered at top speed from France to trains to planes to the saga of Wingrave and Dipstick, not forgetting Mr Bean and all the rest. Then there was no food issue. Daniel arrived and joined in. Poor Jerome must have wanted an early night and managed to extricate himself to see more patients to check on their progress and offer empathy and comfort after his ministrations. Still giggling we let him go…. not before he spied the array of electrical leads in the wall err must be a major grid overload iPad iPhone iMac all essential medical kit you know,' told me.

Oops, I bet he saw my toenail varnish too. Nothing passes that man by.

I thanked him by email: Thank you very much for coming here last evening. We all agreed that piecing together the story of the last two weeks with our own particular brand of chattery humour, is not only funny but of enormous value to the worried * family and groggy patient. There are a few more stories to tell, I sense a blog entry necessary! One thing family do not know† is that a new infection had started the day before. Fortunately, and to my considerable relief cipro is working fast and I'm really OK or statistically 150%? Better than I had ever anticipated at this point. Have a good rest of the week. Thank you very much*

Day 8 home day

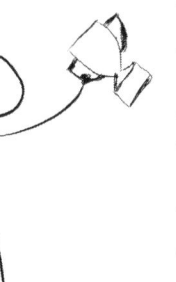

Wednesday, home day. Delighted to beat the pre-op estimate of 14 days…Laden with my hospital-at-home boxes of drugs, Conti pads bags of drugs and products. But with a huge hug to everyone it was time to go.

Hurrah up the M1 and home. Fabulous indeed to be away from the buzzing buzzers to the wonderful own bed. But I admit it, away from all that security all that reliance on professionals, home alone is scary. How to assemble all the drains and bits? How to keep everything clean? Sort out the drugs?

Dry out the night kit?

Assemble the day kit?

How on earth does that connector connect to that one?

One day I will write a guide. I now know the answers and I thought I knew it all last time. But no. How to cut the origami style dressings to fit around and within the catheter. How to stop worrying that the night bag will leak all over the floor. (See entries way back in 2011) Answer: put it in a washing up bowl…simply. How to answer the doorbell without rushing downstairs trailing the catheter bag frame and ALL…. that's another story. And more…. anyhow for now…I'm home I'm sorting it…. I can do it….of course I can. Help. What did they do? So, what did they do? Skip this if you hate the gory details…They as in Wingrave and Dipstick, reconstructed bladder, took down Boari* (*bladder reconstruction to join up to ureter in 2011) …But couldn't get to the old ureter for the right kidney. But have sealed off… and then they used (or as they call it…. harvested and grafted] some of my abdomen to make a kind of parabola[21] to shove. Bladder in to create more tension/pressure which should then graft everything into a more stable place. Very very clever stuff. Main expected outcome is few or no infections. Then all fixed and done. Ta Da!

By Day 10

I had not heard from any clinician since I left hospital. It seemed odd after all that intricate 'tricky' surgery all that amazing, personalised care. Then no one followed up. Did it matter? Perhaps not to the consultants and nurses. They must have to switch to the next patient coming in. Such clever stuff. What an amazing responsibility to take

---

[21] Laparotomy, take down of Boari Flap, division of remaining ureter, colposuspension and autologous rectus fascial colposacropexy (see: www.baus.org.uk).

the trust of that patient into the surgeon's hands. It must be nerve racking. I think if it were me, I'd love to know if all was ok afterwards. Had I made things worse? Better? Too early to tell. Patient ok enough?

Hoping I was doing the right thing I got on with it on my own. Guessing the drugs, dressings, pain control, catheter changes, stands, antibacterial…blah. But I had done it all before. Way back in 2011 I got home after nearly 4 weeks in/out of hospital. One night with my catheter stand by my bed. Catheter day bag linked to catheter night bag which is hung on frame. I slept through the night (thank you painkillers all! I must have dropped a nice book I had been reading on loan from a friend. Daniel was up bright and early for work. As he showered, I realised to my horror, I had left the night bag tap open all night. Brilliant continence sheet had, along with the towel absorbed the whole lot. Fantastic. Smelly soggy but all in one place. Only problem. Was that my loaned lovely book was totally soaked through with smelly pee.

Amazing that it sorts of expanded as it soaked. I stumbled up. Gathered the mess into a bin bag. Taking soggy smelly books too I tentatively get myself downstairs. Stuff bin bag in bin chucked the book in the bottom oven! Having stumbled back to bed, ordered a new copy on Amazon! Phewee. Ages and ages later, I came across the horribly bloated but dried out book. Into the bin went that too. No one ever knew. I think. Hell, whatever could I have said by way of explanation? Anyhow back to now.

Post op days….

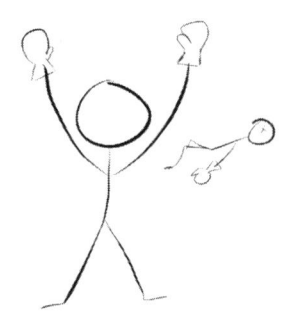

Tuesday 25th District Nurses visited and voiced their concern that too much blood and gore was erupting from the wounds being drained. Suggested should ring a hospital. That I did. Dipstick then rang. Eek they wanted me back in London. Bugger. I saw their radiographer who was brilliant and explained what he had to do. As politely as I could I halted the flow lest things got out of hand. Hang on I said 'I've done this before. Indeed, I already have a suprapubic. That is what you need to inject' with the nicest ever grace he stopped his chat. 'Whoa let's start again. I have no information about you. All I have is *blood in urine*. Economy of words. Well, we all know that one. So, I started again. Explained the saga. I actually gave him a potted account of the last year or so. Not least the revelation that I had a supra pubic! So, the whole procedure equipment etc. had to be changed. Poor man had thought he had a quiet morning. Things got worse when his x rays revealed a missing kidney (forgot to tell him that) also the clear outline of SNS … (forgot to tell him that too) …glossed over the gall bladder bit…and never did explain the metal pins in the spine! Oh dear. Then a scrabble around for a new leg bag. He was utterly charming about it all and admitted he had not yet got used to Dipstick's style of doctoring. I better not tell him he never ever will. Which led me to an NHS England EICC phone call I had yesterday. Talked about the latest draft etc. When I'd finished the NHS senior nurse at the other end asked: 'are you a clinician?'. To which I could only reply: 'hell no, I am only a patient'.

He was great. Funny too.

Saw Wingrave Let's clamp it. That is the valve on the catheter so that my bladder would begin to fill with urine for the first time. Fingers crossed.

OK. I spoke.

Wednesday 26th

Catheter kept blocking, bits and bobs and gore floating about. I tried valiantly to unblock it myself. Gave in. Asked for help. Hospital specialist nurse not in, Wingrave and Dipstick now away, then I remembered the district nurses. They came out. They talked to Dipstick on the phone. Between us we got it going again.

Saturday 29th. Help. Back to square one. Blocked again. Tried nurses. No answer. Must be busy. Text Dipstick. On the number he had given me for the purpose. No response.

Nuttier than usual…. Thu, 03 Sep 2015

I seemed to have appointments in my calendar every day this week with: Surgeon 1 or a Dipstick or radiography. Or even Surgeon 3. Oh, and the dentist too… Confusion reigned for a while. I couldn't remember where, but it turned out neither did anyone else. A 'diary' clash occurred. Anyhow Jerome to the rescue once more. Order restored. Logical plan in place. Early train. 8:03 Top tip: see previous blogs and leave station via hotel.

Visit the loveliest toilets in London. Exit via reception. Porter whistled up a cab from Marylebone Rd. Marvellous. No queues and speedy boarding. Done that a few times in the last few months I …reckon the staff think I'm a long stay guest!! 'Hello'… 'Good morning'…… 'nice day'……… got there 3 minutes late. Ushered to the waiting area. Seats in there look lovely but damned uncomfortable with a sore back. Assume my usual standing pose by the water thingy. Then Dipstick turned up, fired questions at me and pathetically I allowed myself to be ushered downstairs to Amazing Nurse. Aha she says 'I recognise you're famous I Heard you speak …few weeks ago …Battersea Continence Conference….'

Anyhow between us we devised a schedule for the morning truthfully as we admitted to each other we actually had no idea what we were meant to be doing. Cutting a long story short. Gulped coffee and water. Dipstick reappeared and removed the suprapubic. With a mighty tug he did just that and then asked if anyone (me?) could see to the dressing. As no one seemed to move (not least me) he generously suggested he could.

do it himself *'even though I am a surgeon'*?!! Pathetically again I smiled wanly (is that the right adverb?) ….and off he went as I waved goodbye. Hang on I said to his disappearing back…do I need antibiotics?

'Oh yes' he said. 'Has that been organised?'

Hell, as if? Like whom would know? Me? Was I meant to do that?

So top tip 2: make sure to get antibiotics to take home after the catheter is taken out.

Remembering my list of questions 'can I drive'? I yelled over the curtain…. 'Yes' says Dipstick from somewhere …. great in that case I will. Amazing nurse returned. We devised a going home strategy. She gave me a phone in number. Also, to just ring Dipstick… Don't worry about it. No question too silly. Or ring her first and she would forward messages. Good plan. Write a diary, she said. Get into a routine. Ok ok … off we went…we could do this… what was I doing…oh …off to Step once more? Met daughter 2 for quick a soup and a roll with coffee and glass of …water. Top tip 3: Don't drink coffee water and soup straight after the catheter is removed…. Or take a change of clothes. On to train. Top tip 4: sit near 1st to get free Wi-Fi (if no seats sit in 1st and upgrade). Top tip 5: IF you leave your newly acquired gifts for friends at home on the train, by mistake. Ring Lost Property, say it's catheters and a charming man will retrieve it. Dammit. WHATAMILIKE? Frrrrr Top tip 6: when getting into the cab at home-station duck down. Crashing biff on head on door frame. Nearly finished me off! So, I'm Back home …more news soon…I should be thrilled at the fast-paced rate of progress. But actually, even I was petrified. And I am tough.

Excellence in Continence Care Tue, 08 Sep 2015

Lying flat on the floor recovering from my first pain clinic in London. I dialled in to the EICC Programme Board meeting. This unstoppable Board has managed to pull together clinicians and NHS experts to produce a Commissioning Framework. Permission has been granted to proceed to publication. Publication is soon. The group I was involved in is a section on Patient Empowerment. My main concern is the use of language. The awareness of people of all ages of what might be possible to make better, bladder and bowel. No one can find a cure, no one is saying it can be solved. The idea is to improve services. To enable patients to find the help they need in the most efficient manner. That is economic for the CCG[22] and indeed economic in terms of opportunity cost, days lost at work, holidays, quality of life etc. for the patient. Before I started on all this, I honestly thought the word 'continence' meant 'incontinent', old ladies, with leaking

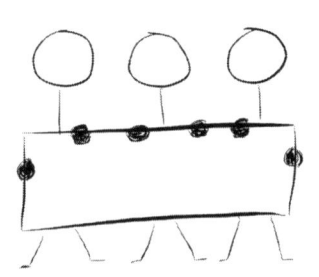

---

[22] Clinical Commissioning Groups (CCGs) commission most of the hospital and community NHS services in the local areas for which they are responsible. Commissioning involves deciding what services are needed for diverse local populations, and ensuring that they are provided. CCGs are assured by NHS England, which retains responsibility for commissioning primary care services such as GP and dental services, as well as some specialised hospital services. Many GP services are now co-commissioned with CCGs. All GP practices now belong to a CCG, but CCGs also include other health professionals, such as nurses. (https://www.england.nhs.uk/ccgs/).

bladders. Some 6 years later I have learnt the word continent is rubbish. That people young old middle aged and adolescent too, may have bladder and or bowel issues. The big taboo. Those issues can be made more bearable by direction to better self-treatment, access to 'continence' products via the NHS and better public awareness. We are talking about long term conditions affecting many people. Melanie Reid in her Times column has often spoken about a need for heightened awareness of the catheter conundrum. An indwelling catheter was invented by a Dr Foley. It was a brilliant idea at the time. However, that was in 1929. Not a lot has changed since then. However, catheter associated urinary tract infections, trauma and overuse, cause big issues for patients. By using better catheters, where possible single use disposable catheters, patients can manage their dysfunction, reduce infection and therefore lower antibiotic use or admission to hospital. It should or could be simple. But there are more complications than that… Until 6 years ago I thought a catheter was a horrid latex pipe from bladder to bag. BUT NO, it does not have to be. There are products out there that mean people can use a small 'mascara' sized catheter to empty the bladder. How great is that. What amazingly clever scientists and engineers are out there finding better ways to improve dignity, self-esteem, confidence and everything that goes hand in hand with that? …. they ARE available. It is just so hard to find out where, how and when. But a big plea from me. Could the experts find better indwelling catheters too? They are just so unsophisticated…it's ridiculous.

Blog entry: You should have seen me blithering around in the middle of the night last week. Bed soaking wet, me soaking wet, trying not to wake D who I suspect was soaking wet but did not realise! Then realising stupid catheter connection was wrong. Could I work out how to correct that? Change the sheets, change me, avoid D…? Rang District Nurses for help. They had a big panic and couldn't get here for two hours. I said not to worry I would set my alarm and just use a leg bag till morning. So that is what I did. Bleurgh.

But I digress, I am so impressed at the 'process', at the way in which the EICC Chair has managed to open doors and gather skills and expertise. The next stage was media communications or comms as they call it. I was involved with that bit. *Don't watch your breakfast TV for a while folks*, I warned. It might just put you off your cornflakes if I appear!

Under My Skin…an ode (aspirational) to spinal implant Wed, 30 Sep 2015

Under My Skin a blog I wrote to explain the 4 sessions of Neuromodulator in preparation for the implant. It took me a year to persuade the local CCG to refer me, even though we all agreed I did not need their approval. Bureaucracy gone nuts. It took a further 6 months to be called to see the consultant. Only to discover I was on the list for the wrong clinic. Thank goodness I was allowed to still be seen. Another 'assessment' by a psychotherapist and specialist nurse to approve me for the programme. So now 2 years on I might be on the waiting list currently running at 18 weeks. I hope I am on it sometime. The MDT meets, then writes to us and copies the GP, once we are approved. So, it could be a while yet. The 4-week programme then, is a good way of keeping the patients off the waiting list but at the same time engaged in the project and testing the resolve to make changes and improvements to pain management. That is cynical but when I chatter to the other 5 the consensus is the same. But I was lucky. Others had waited considerably longer. They had come via Newcastle, Canterbury, Kent, Essex and London. But at least one patient had waited considerably less. It's all about persistence and postcode. Expectations of the NHS are so high. The sheer cost and ongoing expense of such long-term treatment has to be carefully evaluated and those delivering have to be accountable in some meaningful way. I don't know what happens everywhere else. In the USA I guess it would be all insurance claims and ever-increasing premiums. The Obama Healthcare package I gather is making that accessible for those that cannot. Australia always seems to attract young UK doctors. Young doctors newly qualified, my awesome goddaughter is one, and I gather are keen to leave the UK and head to the Southern Hemisphere. Why? The imposition of Mr Hunt's new working contract. But they are our clever kids. The ones who were at the top of their schools. Then we've spent so much on training them for 5, 6, 7 years then…. we make it so horrible they want to take their brains and skills abroad. This was nuts. What could be done to sort it?

So, weeks 3 and 4 of Pain Clinic and the Neuromodulator Programme. Session 3: We were encouraged to think about unpeeling the onion skin layers of our thinking. Why did we react to that situation like that? What are our independent strategies? The ABC Activation Consequence .... Behaviour. Set up the courtroom drama in our heads. What is the evidence FOR our thinking? What is the evidence AGAINST our thinking? Consider our belief systems. Consider the word USELESS: Use – is a function Use Less is psychologically and emotionally unhelpful. Use relaxation to reboot, turn the neuron volume down. Use a flare up checklist and share it with our family and friends. Visualise our island Hold a pebble.

Perhaps pacing is like that cold glass of water full at the beginning of the day. Use it sparingly over the day at the beach. Don't drink it all at once!

Doctors at their best.... Rottweilers on the desk Thu, 01 Oct 2015

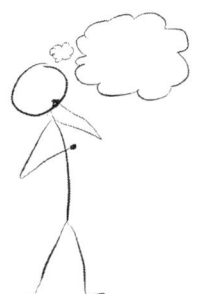

Without going into every tiny detail here is a summary of the last 10 days. Dr Dipstick prescribed a drug to help with the groovy sounding, but so not groovy 'spontaneous voiding'. I subsequently read his clinic letter which referred to a little spasm... Well, if he called that little, I wonder what big was. Spontaneous bladder occurs when the bladder is so full it just empties itself. No warning no ability to stop it and whoosh out it all comes.

Anyhow, I checked the list of side effects with him. Dry mouth he said. I started this new drug. I began to get dry mouth. Fine. Started to get dry eyes. Not fine. Took contacts out. That made blurred vision blurrier… Started to feel faint. Dizzy. Sick. Blood vessels burst in eyes. Rang Specialist awesome nurse. Yikes, she said. Said she would ask Dipstick. As if by magic she called back almost immediately. *Stop the drug.*

Tuesday and Jerome who we have cleverly added to the msu 'form' tells me of uti. Offered assistance. The pain crept up my back reminded me…get sorted ASAP. Wednesday. I tried the GP and the Rottweiler on the desk said I cannot talk to him for 3 WEEKS. Ask if I can talk to ANY GP …. I'll try …. she says. What is the nature of your call? In desperation I say: 'Allergy to drug.' that's only slightly true of course but well it worked. A random GP rang 2 hours later.

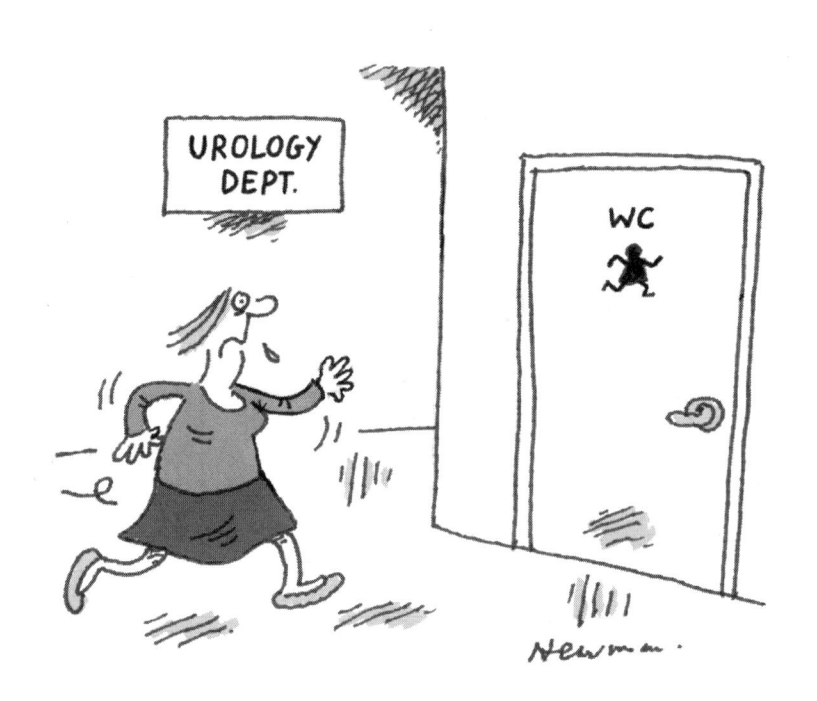

Horse's Arse Thursday 15th

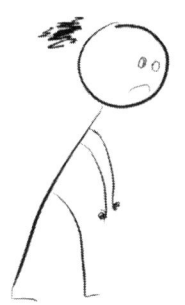

Written on a London pavement. So, I was sitting on a step. I'd rather have been lying down. FFS.

Phone call Wednesday 14th from Dipstick's office:

"Can you be here by 10 not 12:30"

"Sure," I said inwardly, swearing …. rush-hour train, exorbitant fares, overcrowded early trains, at that time of day. I got up 'crack of' to get everything done. Remembering to reschedule my whole day Not a great start to the day, I fell UP the station stairs, coffee splattered everywhere, it stank all day…all that long day actually, as for injuries …. Hip, hand, knee took the brunt of it. So, there I was at the clinic, 'Good news' receptionist said.

'Surgeon is running on time today'.

Hurrah…and I was immediately ushered downstairs. Wearing an invisibility cloak was handy, as I waited patiently, Dipstick was already there. He and a radiologist were chatting about the merits of schools which were single tier i.e., no transition or two tiers, i.e. change school at 11 or 12 or 13…fascinating stuff. Of course, I do actually know a bit about that. But I am 'just-a-patient'. I was scanned by radiologist, but Dipstick just ignored. It's that invisibility cloak again. The radiologist did say he thought my bladder was not emptying well. I knew that really. But at least Dipstick would know the 'real' rubbish from the report too. I went back to waiting room. I just stayed there…. standing, pacing, moving, stretching, wiggling my back, I sat a bit in those horribly uncomfortable chairs, in other words I was in the waiting room, waiting AND waiting AND….. yes, waiting and waiting and waiting and ….

Waiting…

I was there two hours, before I politely asked how long it would be. I was told to allow at least another half hour. So, I said I would get a bit of fresh air outside. So, there I was, and I started to blog to calm down. I also re-re – rescheduled meetings yet again. Bugger. I paced the pavement for a bit. Couldn't stand it inside. So nearly went home. Bloody hell. I think I worked out what had happened. Wonder if I dared ask for a coffee? Every patient in the waiting room seemed to be talking on a mobile. Ignoring polite notice not to use phones, they just merrily chatted away. A bit likes on trains. The contracts I must have heard, the confidential legal advice I've overheard, it's not that I wanted to, the invisibility cloak seems to descend …do they not realise everyone can hear every word?

One patient was clearly a consultant. He was talking to his patient's GP about the mutual patient's gall stones. It sounded like a nice surgical invoice would sort that. Then he spoke to his secretary about unpaid client accounts, he told her he needed to pay some bills. Then he rang his bank for balances, two accounts; one medico legal, the other was his clinic patient account. So, the whole waiting room heard his password *'horse's neck'*… Oh and then he rang a travel agent to book his holiday in Albufeira, Portugal, with a certain Lisa.

We all clocked his name, surname, her name, surname and spelling too! Oh, and he is to be going after half-term with his family, to 'The Sao Rafael Atlantico' hotel on P.E.N.E.C.O. beach. He spelt that out too you see. Despite my efforts to ignore him, read my book and cut out his loud strident tones, he just managed to fill the whole room. What a prat. He got called in… Of course, before me. After all HE IS a DOCTOR Jacq remember you are only-a-patient. I was at that point standing, reading, over by the door, but of course invisibility cloak on, tsk, as usual. A French lady on her phone was whispering which even MORE was annoying than talking loudly… Oh, and a Norwegian lady on the phone. I think she was peed off… from what MJ has taught me of the language. 'Tak'. That's thankyou in Danish, learnt that from the Bridge on TV! In the corner was an elderly couple who talked about their taxi journey which they'd planned to take an hour and a half, but in reality had only been half an hour, so they were early, so next time they would book it later, but the traffic was not too bad, so maybe they should book it later or maybe….arg ghghghgh so it went on …blah at each other so loudly. Their hearing aids must have needed a decibel or twenty changed. Losing the plot, I found that outside …the pavement was nice, quiet even. Got a few strange looks. Said good morning and swiftly got corrected by a very well dressed charming old lady out for a stroll. 'It's Good Afternoon' she said. Silly me.

Later on: I realised my phone which was on SILENT was vibrating, the nice receptionist was ringing… "He's ready to see you now". I cannot explain the consultation. It did not go well. I did try to explain I'd been there a long time he ignored that…. he tried to explain what drug he wanted me to try. We didn't really listen to each other. I didn't ask any of my questions and fought back the tears, angry at myself for allowing the frustrations to get to me. I didn't understand a word he said. He said my bladder was draining well. But I tried to explain I did not agree. Neither did the radiologist. So, he kindly offered to redo scan but that meant waiting for another radiologist, to arrive for the afternoon clinic. So, I said no thanks. I'm sure he thought I was making it up. I couldn't explain anything. It did seem to be my fault. Everything. In addition, he had forgotten about all my allergies. Ooh no need for the allergy protocol. Urodynamic next. Reaction to last drugs? He'd forgotten that too …who cares how crap they make you feel just keep taking the medicine. He shoved a box of tissues at me whilst he dictated his letter. Took me back to the desk, relieved to have gotten me swiftly out of his way. Reception lady queried why I've been there so long. I nodded, bit my lip and said nothing. So, she must've realised. She couldn't book urodynamic because the secretary was 'too busy'! I hate urodynamic so much I was actually pleased. She took my msu form/ sample and said the secretary would ring with result. As if. No chance, I knew that was unlikely.

I so nearly made it to front door to escape, but a lovely brilliant lady on front door reception, (no idea of her name, we always swap a small chat), she made BIG mistake, by being really, really nice. That did it. Tears. Offered a cup of tea. Could've done with that earlier. Said No More tears. Explained the morning to her. She mentioned she would ask patients not to use phones. She suggested I write to the practice manager. I noted his name. Of course, I won't. Finally got away. Trains up the creek. I got home eventually 12 hours after setting off that morning.

POSTSCRIPT: Practice Manager rang. He could not apologise enough. He offered to check urodynamic, msu. He suggested I email outstanding questions to Dipstick. I said no point. Would not get an answer. He suggested I emailed them to him, and he would ensure I DID get the answers. Of course, I did not hear back. Nor will I. ffs what on earth was the point…

- **Sat, 17 Oct 2015 Messages received:**
- **Di**: *I am as sorry as I have only just found time to read this most brilliant ever of your blogs. I so sympathise with you – what a hideously frustrating abomination of a day. What exactly happens to a doctor between the stage when they are moaning about 70-hour weeks and having to emigrate to becoming an overpaid consultant who obviously shares his eating arrogance with the patient(s) sitting right in front of him? Units. We are all units, invisible until legal redress wins an infrequent victory. They get paid whether good or bad or indifferent, why not stick with indifferent? No responsibility in the public sector, NHS. No Hope of Sympathy/Support. D*

- **Patsy**: Dear Girl what a shit day you endured on Thursday. I was almost in tears for you. I can't believe the level of crass incompetence and your patience was unbelievable. I think a strongly worded letter is required…. ….
- **NB says**: This is simply outrageous Jacq what can be done? You/ we must make sure it does not happen again are you by any chance a patient at the London Clinic? If so please tell me We should find out who the Chairman of the Trustees is where you are so badly treated and send him your blog I am sure Daniel would agree Please tell me which is your hospital? Xx N
- **MHR says**: Three things:
- You need a publisher.
- You need another surgeon. STAT!!! Is he the only authority in his field?
- As a now retired litigator highly frustrated with all thing's customer facing in this country, please consider bringing me with you next time. I totally get what you say about being so frustrated and upset that you couldn't get your words/questions out. I had similar issues trying to advocate for my dad when he was ill last year. Surgeons (particularly orthopaedic in my experience) behave like they are demi-Wingrave s and patronise. UGGHHH.
- **SW says**: I can give you back language, holly **** – what are they on? Patient care 1/10 – totally crap – unbelievable – I have had urodynamic

experience x 2 and it is utterly degrading – but I am sure you have been through much worse x 100…. I just wish for your sake just one person was in charge of you and your treatment…. Bloody hell….

Badly Behaved Patients Wed, 11 Nov 2015

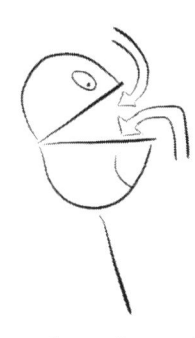

Wonderful, amazing London Teaching Hospital. NHS at its very best. Made lots of new friends, lots of chatter with patients and staff… I'll write it properly when my opiate head clears. My worry though is the expectations of patients. They are rude, demanding and arrogant. Not all but quite a few. I tried to think it through. I'm tetchy sometimes… Like that HorseArse Thursday! BUT, asking for a 'smoke' before going to the theatre? REALLY. Using mobile phones (that old chestnut!) well I mean shouting into the phone and turning the incoming volume up so high everyone else can actually hear both sides of the conversation? REALLY. Asking for painkillers 5 minutes after nurses have just done 'drugs? A niggle to catering though…why can't we have a piece of fruit AND a yogurt?

It's a small thing. They were so amazingly efficient on this oh so specialised ward. But what about trying healthy eating fresh fruit? Salad? A carrot? As for trying to self-catheter whilst lying flat and feeling groggy……generally nurses do not understand the self-catheterisation. Not seen it before. Well, that's another tale... There must be many more stories... I'll think of some more and add. Bet the medics have millions. More of that later... Messages from so many wonderful friends and this from Mel Reid:

- *You are an amazing woman...wishing that things go well for you as my student son said to me when I was in hospital "whatever drugs they offer you, take them. All" MR x*

The Spine Thu, 12 Nov 2015

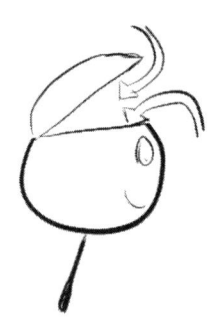

Quite apart from all the bladder bits grumbling away in the background, there has been the spinal nightmare. It seems according to my spinal surgeon, Mr Spine, that the bladder, kidney etc. infections have resulted in a degeneration of my spine. Obviously. Spinal fusion and spinal spacers had been seriously big operations and had made some improvements. But was now getting worse. I refused another fusion. I wrote to appeal to my CCG for referral to London. Cutting a long story short. I got there in the end. I survived the Pain Management Programme and even started a site for the patients. It was called 'under my skin' I am finally and proudly a patient at London Neurology. When I had my consultation with, let's call this Doctor, Mr Hypodermic, he told me he wanted to

   a) Fit a device called a Nevro. HF10. I think. This, he said, has just been licensed. It has high frequency and does not cause paraesthesia (needle sensation).

b) He would do a trial. On the table. And a complete implant, in one single procedure.

c) The Nevro is particularly suited to leg and back pain together i.e., for me a good thing.

The Pain Team and pre-admission clinic staff had told me that there would be a two week trial. The 'paperwork' was promised but never arrived. With some trepidation I made my way as instructed, to the hospital for 8 am on Monday 10. Dear daughter 2. L, offered to come too. Usual domestics completed food, dogs, milk and a full freezer. We giggled our way to London. No seats. I sat on the luggage rack. L on the floor. We swapped commuter stories with our newfound friends as we jiggled and giggled to London.

We checked into the hospital. Worked out which building which ward…thank goodness for without L I would have ended up in the paediatric department.

A flurry of activity and a nurse rushed in, did her admission sheet. Wrist band. Like a boarding card. Surrendered all liquids. Baggage checked and labelled (yes). I was instructed to get into 'gaping-gown' before surgeon arrived… I had been told by the Pain Team that he only does Monday afternoons so NOT Monday mornings Then an Anaesthetist sped in. Turned out he's from our hometown, trained at our hospital.

'Bad luck' I said as we ran through. Asthma? Check allergy? Check meds? Check. He said I would be 'going down' soon. Years of experience …I knew I would not be going ANYWHERE soon. So, I read my paper, read my book, practised my bridge app... Couldn't help but overhear as my neighbour-separated-by-a-mere curtain told her sad story and yelled down her phone. Listened while she insisted on a smoke while the theatre porter waited...... and eventually off she went down...., '.down'.

Still I waited and did another crossword, stood, stretched, lay down, sat, watched Downton on my iPad....and before I knew it, it was afternoon...and a skinny Geeky looking boy, another anaesthetist He too went through the whole asthma? Check allergy? Check meds? Check, again. Immediately followed by none other than the great man himself. Phew. For it was indeed the Mr Hypodermic.

He kindly and clearly explained the plan. 'Trial on the table and then implant straight away, if successful'. I dared not ask what would happen if not. He wielded a big board pen and marked up my back. I signed the indecipherable consent.

He politely congratulated me on still wearing my 'pants'...so good for marking the comfortable spot for battery pack. I could not possibly explain my aversion to the paper variety usually supplied. They go missing, the moment the sniff of gas appears. Let alone the potential for spontaneous voiding so' he said 'we are all ready to go down'...however, much to his disgust, the Houseman had not done the clerking. Whatever the hell that meant I have no idea. A young 12-year-old looking doctor (I must be getting old) nervously approached. Apparently, she was the House Officer. None the wiser I went through asthma. Check. Allergy? Check. Meds? Check. She asked if I'd had any previous operations. Pah…as if! So tempted to say no… I handed her all my own papers…'look' I said, 'how about you take all these and write it up at your leisure'. Her look of relief meant I had said the right thing…so off she nipped dropping papers as she flew.

Oh well. A nurse arrived. 'Quick' she said 'we better go, the Mr Hypodermic is waiting'…. racing through the darkened ward (siesta time lights low!) clutching gaping-gown…we caught a lift. Nipped along to theatres, the manager there sent us packing…wrong theatre! Friggity…back to the lift…giggling. I said, 'oh well let's go for a coffee then'. ….she grabbed me (and gaping-gown) …before I could imbibe and we disembowel (well, nearly) into the basement. The dark nether regions of the great building. We nervously knocked on various gloomy pew green doors. At last, we found the Mr Hypodermic. He was not impressed. I ended up apologising for being late. Why on earth it was me apologising I do not know. However, the Mr Hypodermic swung into action. He was solicitous, positioned pillows, legs, gaping-gown…the lot. See? Keep your pants on patients. It's important. I was fascinated by the sheer number of people in the theatre. They all had a role. They all seemed totally calm, totally in control. Totally wonderfully caring too. Equipment everywhere. Lights from all angles. I'd love to know what it's all for. One day one day I'd love to have a tour with an explanation of just what on earth goes on. A fascinating process, if only it was not me (and gaping-gown). The anaesthetist got started and chatted as he worked, He rammed oxygen up my nose. I really don't remember a great deal. The Mr Hypodermic was chatting away if memory serves me right, he mentioned gin and tonic. The Nevro rep zoomed into my vision with a laptop. Asked me to tell her if I felt anything. She fiddled and twiddled and no I felt nothing. Tried again NO. Eek I was tempted to just say YES, but one more fiddle and twiddle and bloody hell a jolt of sort of electric tingle up my leg. The Right Leg RL…phew…she turned it up a bit and eureka… the Whole Right Leg WRL. Oh, my days it really was working. Yes. WE made it…

The Mr Hypodermic zoomed into view… "I judge by your enthusiastic noise at this end of the table we have success".

I could've hugged the man.

He would hate that though.

Anaesthetists then began to administer and explain the next stage…. glorious wonderful oblivion…. I woke up briefly in Recovery to violent puking. Dearest anaesthetists zoomed in worriedly finding potions to plunge in fast. Descended back.

to glorious oblivion and then awoke up on the ward…found it was 7.00pm and my awesome daughter was already there, waiting for me Pret coffee to hand. YES. D arrived as did BFG all clutching wine gums and fruit gums… Don't remember much more that night. Lovely nurses checking and watching and checking. Other patients all seemed wonderful. One of the patients I later called Lady Edith. She, I recalled, had bounced awake in the bay opposite me in Recovery. My recollection is that she sipped tea 'down there' with a massive bandage around her head as if not a care in the world. \Amazing lady as I later found out. She sprinted off to shower and looked, clutching her brain drain bottle...literally from her head. She came over for a chat and we discussed the label the doctors had stuck on her head bandage. It said, 'flap open'. 'It's the brain' she said. 'Infection after surgery. Got to drain.' Of course. Her husband was under instructions to bring yogurt and fruit for breakfast. Clearly a seasoned patient. Her son brought lunch, a Pret salad. Supper, something a little bit nice from Pret, was brought in by my husband. Nice North London family. We chatted away. Another lady had clearly been their ages, her family came to visit and patiently tried to chat. Nurses sat with her encouraging food. Another, had two small sons who pleaded with her to get better, why are you here? Why are you ill? Why can't you come home? Poor boys. I gave them my wine gums. Daughters of an older lady opposite me scurried in with washing, and fruit parcels and jolly drinks. Wow what amazing strong families these are. The ward ran smoothly. No querying of drugs, catheters, opiates, allergies...as I have grown used to (all those forms before the op!) ... They just so 'got it'. Blooming brilliant. OH, finally, what happened? 'On the table'? Well, the Mr Hypodermic inserted wires into my spine. In the epidural space going up my spine. Then those wires are tunnelled to my left hip (below the pants line!) to a battery which is in a fat-pocket or rather pocket of fat, inside. So, a line of staples to close that bit. Two lines of staples over my spine for the wire bit. Those are sore. No driving. No lifting. No twisting. No swimming. No shower…6 weeks. A lesson from Nevro and Pain Team Nurse Wine, who came to my bedside, spent ages with me, fabulous. They showed me how to charge the battery. Every night like a Tesla car I must charge up for an hour.

There are three points of contact. Seven frequencies, so 21 to try. Wonder if I can in fact try more than one programme. Would that be 21 cubed? Hang on, I better think about my maths…I'll do that. So, Nurse wrote my schedule of changes for me. Gave me my appointment dates. Explained everything. Left phone numbers. Explained what could go wrong and what to do if it did. Nice that. Just so clear. So confident. So, reassuring. At last, I am in the hands of a whole team who know what the hell is going on. They loved the 'Under my skin' site. To say I am delighted with my 'Nevro' is an understatement…After the initial 'wash down' the stimulator seems to have switched off the pain in my leg. That is utterly stupendous. I cannot tell you how much that means to me it is like massive migraine has been dulled. Thank you one and all. I know this is only the start. We were warned it is a long process and now we are 'wedded' we are told to the hospital for life. They will check us, challenge us, and calm us. Wow. I really have got that implant under my skin. It has only just been licensed for use. Up to now patients have used an SCS stimulator a bit like my bladder SNS. I.e., the frequency can be felt.

Most patients have to have a two-week trial before full implant. Some end up having an op for the start of trial. Another for the end of the trial. Then 6 weeks later, another operation for a full implant. Not me. Thanks to Harris. I....thank him so very much.

Messages:

- *Amazing Jacq... did not know whether to laugh or cry. So did both. Your sense of irony is the stuff of great theatre, by which I mean Bernard Shaw, not hospital... You also have a new career as a blog site. How utterly wonderful and cool you are. So much love and congrats xx BEE*

Thu, 19 Nov 2015 Brighton

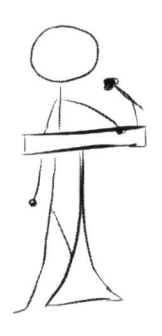

I was honoured to be invited to speak about a subject close to my heart at the Brighton BAUN Conference. As teachers we are trying hard to catch up with the informed evidence-based practice clinicians in the NHS demonstrate. The BAUN conference certainly demonstrated that in spades. I was asked to present the ISC Nurse of the Year award at the Gala Dinner. Such an honour and amazing stories of amazing nurses.

I was also honoured to be invited to attend the All-Party Political Group (APPG) Continence meeting at the House of Commons on Wednesday 18th November. Hosted by Mr Hypodermicess Greengoss, this was attended by NHS England Excellence in Continence Care Board (EICC). This board for which I am Patient Advocate, announced and explained new guidance: Practical Guidance for Commissioners, Providers Health and Social Care staff and information for the Public... Sarah Elliott Chief Nurse, NHS England (South) led on this. In addition, Dr Clare Gerada former chair of the Royal College of GPs and Partner at the Hurley Group, spoke on how CCGs and GPs should implement the new NHS England Guidance on Continence Care. Finally, the Chief Medical Officer Professor Dame Sally Davies was represented by her team who presented the CMO Report on Women's Health. Crucially this report, which is due to be published in December, has a whole section on continence. The next focus will be on women 50-70, so again this will have parallels. The overwhelming evidence from all those who spoke and the many eminent clinicians, was that continence is not just basic but actually an essential area for CCGs, GPs and the general public to raise awareness, improve education and resources, finding ways to ensure that this is a non-negotiable area to be addressed across the country. I am only a patient, but my impression is that all those present felt that this was a well overdue initiative which demanded immediate action with measures to ensure compliance and accountability attached. The guideline can be found on the NHS website, and it also includes a small section of my own story.

Bladder in Brighton...behind the scenes Thu, 19 Nov 2015

Here is an informal take on the week: Was honoured to speak at the Brighton BAUN Conference. Fabulous room, sea view, fell asleep on arrival in the ginormous bed. Woke up to find I was already late for dinner....Sat next to a lovely Italian Urological Surgeon on the top table. Oh, my days ...my 'Tourette's'...if I said 'peed off 'once I said it 100 times. Fabulous and worthy prize winner. Tourette's moment as I announced the prize I said: 'Fantastic and worthy winner...she managed to overcome the hassles of admin for her patients by using simple communication methods...i.e., mobile phones to avoid the gatekeepers of phone call centres...I then said: 'Wonderful a lady after my own heart, cut the crap...get it sorted'. The raucous laughter was not worthy of the words uttered.

I left the dancing guests and went up to my room for an early night, not least because it takes an hour to charge up the new spinal device each night...the Nevro....it is great and will be hugely better once the 72 (apparently) staples are removed from my back. But the wild November waves were better than any medical intervention through the night. My speech, the next day, was 'My story'. Technical support made it a seamless and easy performance. I showed Sir Lancelot Spratt as suggested by Jerome. It went down a storm and my Tourette's moments? I swore twice and said 'peed' off 50 times. I also met a nurse who had originally programmed my SNS and who had attempted to do my annual check-up last year via Jerome. I met and was invited to co-author a paper for the Munich European Urology Conference in March. After the conference I stayed with Patsy overnight. I was so well looked after. She has another chemo session on Friday. She and I went for her pre-chemo-testing to the amazing groovy and new Pembury Hospital. It is like an airport. I was staggered at the technology and attempts to avoid human interaction. The Rottweiler on the desk reminded us why robots might be better. I was staggered at the ridiculousness of Phlebotomy in a cupboard with no windows, Oncology, in a corner at the end of a long stairway and corridor. Again, NO windows. Nothing on the walls (but Patsy is going to donate pictures). Who is the architect? Wingrave knows they need a patient perspective for goodness sake.

I was honoured to be invited to attend the All-Party Political Group (APPG) name plates, microphones and very serious faces. Well, I tried. I made myself scribble 'do not swear' on my notepad. Patsy had been training me well! Then the eloquent Dr Clare Gerada mentioned a Prof Lee (I think that was the name). Apparently, this highly regarded Consultant in times gone by, insisted on demonstrating catheter usage by dropping his trousers and performing said task to show his trainees how it was done... hah!

Then it was my turn to speak. What do I say ...? To speak...err...err...' I am a catheter user, but I will not be dropping my trousers....'

Dr G interjected: 'oh do oh do'...

Hah I said: 'OK then'.

...dear reader...I DID NOT I promise you faithfully I so did not. I think Mr Hypodermicess was ok with the banter. It was amazing to be there. My various devices only caused a slight scare as I encountered security. We will be going to media soon, my meeting with BBC postponed as Paris horribleness and Junior Doctors in trouble, takes precedence and rightly so. My bladder managed the whole meeting and I so nearly made it without embarrassment ...I do recall asking the CMO delegates to send her i.e., Sally my very best wishes and an x. You see I used to rent a room in her house after we had met in Madrid...that is a very long story that one.

And so, to home and my own bed...I actually slept most of the next day...my body was not keeping up with my brain. Meanwhile, I had learnt so much. Not least that this would be a huge leap forward. The various agencies are working together to make a difference, not working in isolation. Trying to overcome the silo effect of healthcare. In addition, 'patient voice' i.e. Jacq was mentioned. Bet they wished they had someone more polite.

Messages:

- *From P:* J If this is not already a blog it needs to go online. So, get on with it – nothing else to do, after all!! P
- *From G*: Good morning J – thanks so much for a splendidly irreverent read which contained so much critical learning for all in the Continence world. I was challenged by a '4' showing on the alarm clock this morning as I headed to Edinburgh for an NHS Scotland review meeting,

and you made me laugh out loud in a very quiet Heathrow. Have a lovely weekend recharging and do send me any link to any 'official' blog you may be putting online. Kindest regards

- **From M:** *Great writing. Love the Prof Lee story! LM*

Fifty shades Fri, 04 Dec 2015

Another Urodynamic test, or a whiter shade of pale as I have called it before. This time I have to self-pay …a long story. Nice little hospital St Johns Wood. Close proximity to the huge hospital for spine surgeon Mr Economy -of-Words. Scene of the original bagel clutching blog. Confusion at reception directed to the wrong place despite my protestations. Of course, only the patient would know that. Told to drink tons of water…. wasn't expecting that. Found surgeon in the end. Yikes really late. Hoping not too annoyed ended up apologising for my tardiness. He was on the phone and explaining to whoever was on the other end that he'd taken someone else's coat by mistake (!), then a bit of medicalness for sorting so hopefully I'd not actually held him up too much. Nice nurse. Nice chatter with fellow patients outside. We compared our awesome gowns. Why can they not be designed to be Velcro sticks? Leaping in and out of the bathroom clutching gaping gowns we managed to avoid too many odd looks from passers-by. One porter cleverly avoided eye contact every time he passed. Anyhow Dipstick was lovely, considerate and matter of fact. Tipped the X-ray thing and I upside inside out, hung on, stopped me falling off the damn thing. Results next. I will discuss the results the following week…

Saggy Bottoms 13 December 2015

The Urodynamic had been the previous week. Fifty Shades of Pale Day. As we were short of time that day, Dipstick said he would go through the Urodynamic results at our next consultation. He asked me to check with his secretary that I did have an appointment booked and that SNS Rep would be there. I did. It was not. It got sorted. Soooo arriving at a good time for a confirmed scheduled appointment at 11:45. Imagine my thoughts as I took in the scene at reception. Dipstick had his head in his hands and was muttering, the reception lady looked faint… *'You are so NOT going to like this'* said Dipstick to me.

It turned out that Mr SNS, the supplier rep, was running very late, uncertain of arrival time. Dip needed to get to theatre, medical that is, not West End! Anyhow, they assured me of the absence of mobile wielding loud mouthed patients in the waiting room. (So, they HAD read my letter) I refused the offer of the waiting room. I wandered off to take sanctuary in a coffee bar. As agreed. To await their call for a decision on what to do next. Nearly an hour later, I wandered back to say I could not wait any longer. Receptionist reported that Mr SNS was indeed in the house. I waited. Eventually was called in. Mr SNS wanted to know who had sanctioned the new Neuromodulation Programme. Query interaction with SNS. That got dismissed, with me sort of mumbling away about how I'd tried to get Dip to talk to the Harris. Why the hell I try I do not know. So, Mr SNS suggests having a go with both devices and see what interference there is. Another appointment in a few weeks. Then that was that really. No need to discuss Urodynamic apparently as we had done so already. When? I've no idea. Letter dictated. New msu for the ongoing infection. But I never hear the results. More money to pay …for once I queried it. Urodynamic cost £497 hospital £ 500 for consultant and £180 for follow up fee? I felt it was just an open cheque book. If it were my car in for a service, I'd query it. But somehow, it's unseemly to query bills for my body. No one was available. I did see an awesome Nurse Downstairs. She was fab.

In other news. Christmas Dinner Charity do at the invite of CJC, Lady Taverners. Mary Berry and Jenny Eclair the entertainment. Putting the 'eclair' into the 'berry' or we wish they had. Food was terrible. 450 ladies' lunches returned to the kitchen. Oops. Considerably distracted Angela Rippon kept referring erroneously to saggy bottoms. As all Berry aficionados know it is soggy bottoms. Not of the urological kind. I will try and draw an appropriate cartoon. Too many ladies for too few toilets. So, seeking to avoid any soggy (!) moments four of us went to the male toilet. But emerged from our cubicles to find a solitary man having a peaceful pee. Oops. His embarrassment palpable as he stood frozen, willing us to leave. Ah well we did. Bloomin – bladder!

Happy Christmas Fri, 18 Dec 2015

Happy Christmas…have a wonderful indulgent relaxing fun filled time whoooo.

Behind the scenes…Sun, 03 Jan 2016

We took Christmas to Scotland and saw the flooding at first hand. A miserable time for many. Goodness knows how people cope, recover and restart. What about all those with medical needs? It must be a nightmare. As for the media: TV was ok they filmed for two hours and showed about 1 minute of me gabbling and washing hands. So then, as the BBC had scheduled, home we went for the appointed interview. My mind is not on it. My plan for hair, smart outfit etc. thrown by the lack of time…but arrive BBC did, and they were so nice. Picture the scene: in my bathroom cameraman, lights, hairy microphone thingy and the journalist… My bathroom was too small, so we moved into BFG's. I'm proud of his Father Christmas loo paper that made it into shot. . .

Radio: we were on our way back from Scotland. Stayed in flooded Cumbria. Heard dramatic stories of water filling from the floorboards up and more such horrible disasters. We witnessed for ourselves the sandbags and M6 'lake', so miserable. Atmosphere in the pub on our way home was fabulous. Such stoicism in adversity…even joking about the 'Lake District'. We managed a 'With Nail and I moment! Amazing locals were jam-packed into the pub. The landlady said it was the busiest night of the year.

Interview Day dawned:

No phone signals. Found landline. Sandbags outside! Rain lashing down. Dogs in breakfast dining with us. Long story!

Come morning at 8:00 am and my scheduled interview at 9:30, I realised my mobile signal had disappeared along with the floods …no phone signal. So, I rang the BBC producer using the pub landline, and spoke to the publican…. The interview ended up on landline in breakfast room, surrounded by dogs, coffee, bacon, toast, sausages …and ME…trying to answer open unplanned questions while remembering to repeat my three 'rocks' bladder bowel itspersonal. It was funny in retrospect but stressy in reality! L telling me to take the call upstairs in my room ….me gesticulating that actually I was already 'ON AIR' D munching toast, dogs pouncing on any dropped crumbs…. rrrr I'll never be a movie star…

Messages

Bee wrote I wish all this background information had made it into the 'shots' and 'talk space' for the general public, for added piquancy. It makes it all the more impressive. How did you concentrate and appear so unflappable and unflapped? You will be a movie star, says the fairy.

God mother xx.

- the program when I get home. A brave thing to do and I really admire your open attitude. You will help a lot of people. Love p xx.

LETTERS PAGE THU, 31 DEC 2015

The reasons for going 'public' are best explained through the humbling responses… Subject: *Pleased to hear your message on BBC Radio 4 Today programme yesterday (28/12/15) morning.*

- *As a faecal leakage sufferer for 8 years, I was very pleased to hear that your organisation is advocating more openness about incontinence and the possibility of managing and/or treating the condition. I have tried in my own small way to do this, but it is difficult because it's been such a taboo subject. Thank you, very much, and good luck, with your campaign which I fully support.*
- *Have just listened to your radio interview. That was fantastic. What an interview!*
- *You did so well, a wonderful, moving, humourist, informative and giving a very positive message. The interviewer was good too. His inputs were all very appropriate and in no way hog the listener. It was really good.*
- *Yes you are right there "…no one would know…." That you were in a pub, two dogs…"*
- *B: Hello lovely lady, wow what can I say, your to appearance was just fabulous and he will do SO much for awareness. As a fairly young person, I used to find it such a difficult subject to discuss. I've actually had continence issues since I was a child, but the "stigma" stopped it from ever being discussed.*

- *J your story and how you've coped is truly inspiring and you breathe off fresh air!! What you've done will share so much awareness and is just awesome! Thank you thank you thank YOU!! I hope you've had a lovely Christmas whilst fitting in television appearances!! How are you finding the NEVRO? Let's meet up soon, I miss you and our inappropriate humour!! Lots of love xxxxx*
- *A: Think of the inspiration and help you have given strong to people who have never dared to discuss and are constantly worried about*

Try again …bogus Sat, 23 Jan 2016

Monday, Tuesday was teaching, meetings about meetings and fiddling about with a 3-minute presentation which seems to have taken 300 hours to prepare.

Wednesday, I had begun to lose the plot and started to cancel the rest of the week. I made it to the NHS England progress meeting. Not sure I contributed at all as I just could not stop shivering. Friggity. I made it home to be greeted with a line-up of colleagues needing alterations to bloody presentations. Frrrrr. Slept with fleece on, drugged up and knocked out!

Saw the new GP let's call her 'Gladys'. She told me I had an infection. "NO? Really?! Me?! Never. SHER-LOCK. Didn't feel able to share the details. Stupid patient doesn't need that info. I tried to explain I had been on 'Nitrofurantoin' and 'gentamicin' all week. Tried AGAIN to explain I needed to see the lab report. I was so pewky and was struggling to keep stuff down. She said she'd write a script for something stronger and 'special'. Guess what was on her script? 'Nitrofurantoin' arghhhh I just meekly accepted as I had an ace up my sleeve…. That is, Jerome had promised a script. Got that from chemist.

2. Bellini breakfast, Tue, 02 Feb 2016

A week that was: I did some 'emergency' maths support in school. The Head teacher had asked me if I could help with some teaching. Oh yes, I said (do I never learn?). I was teaching Monday Tuesday.

Wednesday: Two of us, conference speakers, drove to Heathrow. We negotiated a bizarre check-in clerk. Security caused a kerfuffle my various implants always caused a fuss. I had agreed to a private search. Tsk. Two security guards to accompany me to the little cupboard of a search room. All it was, was a pat down. I found my fellow speaker; she was ordering breakfast in the champagne bar. Thinking it would be rude not to I joined her. Bellini and fruit salad were what we had. Then off we went to Scotland. It was a good conference. Great company. Great speeches. Wonderful hilarious upgrade to another hotel for a few of us including me. Whoop. We laughed like drains as we sipped night caps. A colleague's hilarious tale of euphemisms developed by her boss surgeon: it was called the Roast Chicken story. Conference next day went well. Every speaker had to get 'roast chicken' in somewhere? Very funny. Even made it onto Twitter. Then it was flight home. I slept most of way not least because the next day, Friday, was a teaching day. I crawled home at lunchtime after that and could not move. That week tanked up on adrenalin gent and antibiotics finally caught up with me.

3. BLADDER AND BRAIN STILL NOT IN UNISON

I ended up, inevitably, spending a few days in hospital, thanks to Jerome, to restore bladder. Then it was the final week of term. Parent-teacher consultations were booked for me in my (hospital) absence. I'm thinking doctor's surgeries might be similar. After a full day of teaching, we all started school by 7.00 am. Although on that day the school nurse sent me home at 12.00. With high blood pressure and a massive headache, I went home. I showered. I catheterised. Instilled gentamicin. Having changed in to 'meet the parents' suit ...I returned to school.... the day ended at 9pm with the last parent talked to, reassured and smiled at.

4. House of Cards, Sat, 16 Apr 2016

This was the day I was in Warwick for a sales rep conference. The delegates all worked for a continence product supplier. Dinner was buffet and team building. The age-old marshmallows and spaghetti task we have used so often in schools! In the morning I did my talk. The audience were 100% receptive. Their laughter at my initial funny story about dipsticks, fuelled my confidence. Then it was a train to London taking the respite for a power nap …. I arrived in London to make my way to the House of Commons. Once through the airport style security, as ever, succumbing to a full search, eventually, me, my bag and case were reunited. The stimulators, chargers, syringes, catheters all caused a bit of a fuss. As ever. Then I made my way into the bowels of government. Two rooms to make Laws and 28 rooms to entertain in! We were in one of these, for The National Continence Care Awards. Or as Daniel kept quipping: 'the bladder of the year Oscars'. Mr Squeezy App[23] was there winning the Technology for patients' award. I met the inventors, they were great. There was much merriment as I told my story of erudite professor of education and her husband's enthusiasm for the app. I was awarded the Patient Champion Award. Our local MP was there

---

[23] Squeezy App. The NHS endorsed pelvic floor exercise app. Developed by Health Tech company. Living With (https://www.livingwith.health/) and Myra Robson physiotherapist. (https://www.squeezyapp.com/)

to meet me and take me onto the balcony over the Thames for the photographers. It was a very good occasion.

5. NICE Guidelines

At the beginning of 2016 I had been persuaded to apply for and succeeded in joining a committee which was to refresh NICE Clinical Guidance on Women's Urinary Incontinence (UI). In addition, the guideline was to establish guidance for women's pelvic organ prolapse (POP). The media attention surrounding the latter was phenomenal. The National Institute for health and Care Excellence (NICE) committee consisted of senior clinicians, three patients and a huge team of researchers. The team met in the Royal College of Obstetricians and Gynaecologists (ROCG) in Regents Park. The pressure and concern over the guideline meant many emails, meetings, overnight stays in Regents Park and teleconferences by the dozen. Due to the nature of the work, I was unable to explain details to my friends and family. It was an experience I found intellectually demanding. I was thrilled to be there to join the rigour, the analysis and attention to detail as we poured over the evidence base. Back at home I was still teaching year 7 and 8 children on the temporary emergency cover I had agreed to do. I was also on the steering group of a teacher research group. I found it increasingly difficult to fulfil my teaching commitments such as they were. With heavy heart I made the decision to 'retire' from teaching altogether. The school had been supportive, understanding and had become a massive part of my life. But I just was not reliable enough my health was not improving.

6. Auf Wiedersehen, Thu, 21 Apr 2016

A brief blog after I had returned from a trip to Germany:

I thought (idiot) I was just speaking for part of a 30-minute slot with other patients. I thought I would hear some interesting debate from policy makers, health and social care providers, NGOs and medical experts on continence care. I thought I would learn a lot. I thought I would see a bit of Berlin, read my book, take it a bit easy after a busy week last week and agent /cephalexin[24] double act to keep me upright. Well... I was very wrong. I did listen to lots of mainly interesting debate from some very clever folks. I spoke far more than 30 minutes. I spoke on film, I asked questions, I disagreed, I agreed, and I agreed to disagree. I did not see Berlin. I did not see my book. I did, however, see many naked men! I walked into the sauna by mistake. Apparently in Germany no swimsuits are worn, and it is unisex. HONESTLY!! I beat a hasty retreat pretending to check the time on my non-existent watch. I did see a beer Keller and vast amounts of pork, sausage, and cabbage. The hotel toilets were awesome, plentiful and had sound effects of twittering birds. I made many new friends and talked far too much. For the most part my new friends shook off the pitying looks and sad faces as they introduced me as the 'patient'. I knew I had made it to the ranks of normal

---

[24] Cephalexin – an antibiotic one of the groups known as cephalosporin.

colleagues when they 'took the pi**'! Yes, all the old jokes still get wheeled out, but this time …. the Chair, Co-Chair and their gang walked back to the hotel from the evening reception at the Beer Keller. To their utter amazement, remember folks, this is a continence conference, they found a MALE catheter on the pavement. Took a photo. Found me, then to the amusement of all there gathered, giggled their glee…. 'Jacq' they giggled 'this must be yours!' Those of you who know me well, will remember that part of my 'story' is to explain a male catheter is needed for installation of gentamicin. (Because the male catheter is longer and thus easier to use with a syringe). Argh. Anyhow, of course, the word soon got around, the story got bigger, and the photo got tweeted. NO, it was NOT mine!! of the 3 patients, 1 carer and 350 delegates from across the world…let alone the residents of Berlin, someone uses a male catheter, in addition to me!

What was the conference outcome? How about a move to patient centred, value driven, guideline adherent service design? How about giving value to patients and their carers? What about thinking about patients as thinking talking responsible PEOPLE. By the way I am not your patient. I am a patient of my doctors. But just because you are a doctor in a roomful of doctors does not give you the licence to call me a patient nor look pityingly at me.

One nurse chose to challenge my assertion that Health Care Professionals do not have mandatory training in continence care.

I KNOW that is true. The ensuing presentations of data PROVED that was true. That is exactly the point. We will never agree if you never believe us. Do not judge your patient...LISTEN to her. Why on earth do we not consider opportunity costs? The cost of poor-quality care, reduction in economic terms of work hours for patients and or carers, let alone quality of life, leisure time and overall contribution to GDP? Why do we not integrate health and social care? pads get funded by social care, catheters by health care. But if you need both? God forbid anyone from either service ever actually TALKS to each other. Let's take that a step further...If I was a diabetic, I would get my needles, syringes and dipsticks on prescription. As I am not a diabetic. I am not allowed to get them on prescription. In fact, I must order and pay for them myself through the chemist. Nor am I allowed a 'sharps' box. As a tearful lady in the chemist last week explained. She too is not a diabetic. She is awaiting surgery of some sort. She cannot go to work. She is on benefits. She cannot get any of these either. There is a theory we can go to the drug addicts' centre in town and get our sharps boxes there.

Yes, we have an ageing population. Yes, that will cost us. People are living longer because they get good care. BUT the overall effect is to move GDP from only 1% to 2%. But what is a HUGE issue is the astronomic cost of bad care which becomes ACUTE care. I ranted: Let us stop the rot NOW. Intervene early. Prevent and 'cure' may not be possible, but quality of life is . . . . . . Just in case anyone was in any doubt I added: My aim is to make bladder and bowel assessment and treatment, a mandatory module in the education of all Health Care Professionals. Medical Schools, Royal College of Nursing, Midwifery…everyone else…it should be as basic as a blood pressure assessment.

7. Open for business 24/7, Sat, 07 May 2016

As I began the wind down of my teaching career, the school exam season was in full force. The May Bank Holiday weekend, as ever, filled with… work. Many papers to mark, moderation to perform and students to chase. Of course, with some parallels to Junior Doctors, teachers 'only work 5 days a week'. 9 till 4 or in our school 8 till 2:30. Which sort of assumes no preparation, before or after. AS IF. I'm guessing our government ministers assume doctors just wander onto the wards miraculously knowing what to do straight away.

With work pressures at home, I had been trying since March to arrange appointment with Dipstick. As ever the pathetic patient knows nothing, does nothing and therefore is nothing. He even sent a rare email suggesting I organise some medicine with the 'girls'. Not sure which girls he meant – bet whoever they are not keen to hear that descriptor. Needless to say, no one had a clue. I decided to give up asking for an appointment or in fact for anything. It was too stressful, and I was always in the wrong. I petulantly wrote to him by email to explain that. The response was an instruction to his office to 'sort it out'. It would not be, because no one not even the 'girls' would have any idea what he wants. Fully aware he was a good I am sure indeed a brilliant, surgeon. He just needed a diary, a PA and an email software package.

8. On it like a car bonnet, Sun, 15 May 2016

I in fact had an appointment with Dipstick but no-one had told me. As I was only the patient, it really did not seem to matter. Obviously, I had had nothing better to do than go to appointments at a moment's notice. Let alone give my employers any notice. NHS Consultants, Jerome tells me, need to give 6-week notice.

That week I also had an appointment in London, with Montmerency- Consultant Microbiology: His swanky office on the third floor meant he clod hopper-ed down all the stairs, in his motor bike boots, to meet and greet me. Then we clomped back upstairs swapping inane banter as we went. I told him Jerome has a cartoon of them both on a motorbike. He laughed hugely over that. We also had this idea of sipping very cold champagne on the roof terrace. Of course! Subsequent emails included Jerome. The banter I cannot possibly repeat but champagne, car bonnets, blankets and more, made sure we must've all been LOL, on our respective trains, or motor bikes home.

Montmorency put forward his plans: *Decided for the 6-week potion idea. Think of your bladder like a 50-year-old (so generous is he!) Teflon frying pan. Needs a recoating. Just do it. Decide. GET ON WITH IT.*

Meanwhile despite a frustrating time on the Dipstick front I had major success elsewhere. My saintly GP sourced NHS magic potions for bladder instillations recommended by Montmerency. I could not thank him enough for constantly sourcing and sorting. He even helped me sort out my sore neck, using his secret 'how-to-get past the Rottweiler trick'.

The next day was Friday: 7.00 a.m. I was back to London. The station staff must imagine I am a commuter bustling up and down to London for my awesome important job. Anyhow, I made it, a bit late to a North London Hospital. Northern Line had been evacuated. There were no trains on the underground. I found a bus. The hospital, once I got there, were wondering where everyone was! They were great.

They gave me a thorough kidney check-up. Headache building and uti brewing I made my way home once more.

9. I'll try not to kill you this week, Mon, 30 May 2016

I had managed to get the magical 'Teflon' installation recommended by Montmerency. But alas another infection bug (ger), had hit. I had trailed into London on the commuter train. To be told to go back home, collect my overnight bag (drugs, chargers for the stimulator, toothbrush etc) and be admitted for IV antibiotics. That was actually a good idea and strangely a relief. Dipstick did not know where I live, it all took a bit longer than he anticipated. His secretary finally gave me the go ahead at 5pm and I was admitted by 7.00pm. IV went in. Cups of tea in and I was asleep in seconds. Morning dawned. Dipstick bounced in. Daniel popped in and said hello and he commented that I looked 'flushed'. Daughter texted, 'I'll bring a coffee over this morning'. The next IV bag went up.... I do not remember a lot after that. Lots of nurses and doctors ran to my bedside. Oxygen mask was rammed onto my face. Heart whatsit monitors stuck onto my body...then so many drips, injections and God only knows what else. My daughter came bouncing in announcing 'coffees' but stopped and whispered as she took in the scene. poor her. The long and short of it was that I was allergic to yet another antibiotic. X-rays and ECG were done and verified I was ok enough. Jerome came, to distract. We thought Black Box[25] thoughts. Calm was restored with constant monitoring, antidotes, and oxygen.

Then it was bank holiday, all doctors-maintained radio-silence, hoping they must be having a nice holiday somewhere I realised not a lot would happen for a while… Having no idea what the plan was for the week ahead I just sort of made it up. But I was only the patient, it really did not matter, or did it?

---

[25] Black Box Thinking Syed, M. (2015). Black box thinking: Why most people never learn from their mistakes—But some do. Penguin.

10. Whitehall, Sat, 04 Jun 2016

June 3rd, 2016, and the next EICC meeting was in Whitehall at the Department of Health. A meeting full of energy the National Grid could surely benefit. Those around the table I held in such esteem. So much had happened quickly and steered skilfully by our chairperson. Sad to say she was now retiring. The note I penned went like this: Thank *you for chairing this amazing group – you have been utterly inspirational. I remember the first time I met you. At the House of Commons dinner. You fend off negativity from those gathered round with such dignity. I have you in mind every time I encounter a stroppy person. The solution… Bat it back. You did. Thus, the EICC was formed if you cannot beat them. 'Join them'. Our first meeting I blogged something about the scary efficient chairperson. Since then, I am glad to say I am not scared of you and certainly have enjoyed many giggles. Thank your awesome lady. Very best wishes for whatsoever you are about to do next. Never say goodbye, it is always…see you soon.*

11. Paper curtains with the fabulous Melanie Reid, Sun, 05 Jun 2016

Extract from The Times of London: Melanie Reid *'I was an incontinent no-show at a continence conference.*[26]

What black irony is that? A "Melanie Reid in her article in the Times this week. '...The ACA is a brave band of health professionals who strive to tackle the universal curse of incontinence. This is a real Cinderella branch of medicine. Few want to fund research, revolutionise treatments or develop 21st-century solutions............. "'The paper curtains in Accident and Emergency in Edinburgh, I noted grimly, were the same as the ones in Glasgow. Bright blue, stiff pleats. Must be an NHS job lot, I reasoned. Lying on the trolley waiting for the consultant, swallowing panic. I was getting too practised at this....

---

[26] Melanie Reid. The Times https://www.thetimes.co.uk/article/spinal-column-a-bladder-emergency-m6jgzdx6c.

12. Stormy weather, Sat, 11 Jun 2016

Weather of the week sort of reflected the mess I got myself into by Wednesday. I was on a weekly, for 6 weeks, treatment of Teflon type stuff to line the 50-year-old frying pan as described by Montmorency. Well Week 1 was a wipe out, as another infection raged, and antibiotics reacted. Week 2 was done in hospital but some weird asthma stuff issues afterwards. Sensibly Week 3 was to be again in hospital and with due care. and attention. Only trouble was that never did get booked, I spent the week cancelling half term plans and waiting, asking, and waiting. ...nothing happened, nothing explained. Worse than that, got told 'things have to be arranged' what things? That is what I dreaded...that feeling of the need-to-know basis that really gets to me. 'You-are-only-the-patient – IDIOT'. which signalled yet another stay in hospital for Week 3 treatment. Only trouble was it had been booked as an 'operation'. Why? no one really could explain.

On admission, the nurse did the usual pre-operation preparation. Rings, nail varnish, gown, paper pants. Asked who the anaesthetist it was or will be etc... You know the form, she looked pityingly when I said I really don't think we needed to do all this. *There there dear.... shhh*...what the hell do you know you-are-only-the-patient. With a rising sense of panic, I made sure I had those a miserable grey papier Mache pewk bowl to hand, oh and I was NIL BY MOUTH for the 'operation' when had I last eaten drunk??? Etc. etc. I jumped to my feet, to see Wingrave, appear. '.Hi. Heard-you-were-here'. His quick-fire social banter evaporated as poor old Dipstick arrived. Looking even more exhausted than ever, green about the gills ready for the sick bowl too. Then they both started firing questions at me. 'Why are you here? 'said Dipstick. 'Bloody good question' I muttered. Dipstick got the confused nurse sorted, explained it is not IN 'theatre' but here IN 'situ' that he would Instil. Did that. Asked me sympathetically if I was ok...? Well, the dam burst. I told him exactly why I was not ok, why continually not telling me what the hell was going on, why continually changing plans on a day-by-day basis, was not only frustrating, but utterly disruptive, mentally, and physically. To me, to my family, my work, everything. I yelled at him and asked him why he had even asked me why I was there, that he had complained (earlier) that he had had many calls about my allergic reactions. He replied: ever so quietly 'I was trying to be informal I do not mean it.' I asked how on earth anyone could get hold of him: Not even the hospital. That they had told me to ring 999. That is ridiculous he agreed. But 'just ring me he said...'ring my mobile'. I could not stop I ranted on long I think the poor nurse was about to start crying too. I rarely let go rarely lose it that this time had probably been brewing for years...it went on and on. He was utterly brilliant after that. He came back to make sure I was 'still alive' I got THAT joke! Several times. He met my youngest two who glowered at him...eek. He came back the next day. He was good. More than that we together made a sensible workable plan for the following week. He even remembered to tell his secretary. He even reminded me to phone him if I needed to. As if.

13. M.B.E. Motivational Brave Educational Melanie Reid, June 2016

Times extract: Melanie Reid has far worse to cope with than me and the extract below is her take on life. Disabled as she is and I am not in any way in her predicament, I totally agree with the sentiment applied to patients i.e., people, everywhere: *The Times 11 June 2016.Melanie Reid Spinal Column: That's the trouble. Everyone thinks disabled people must be handled like unexploded bombs, and it is not good for our reputation as a tribe, or as individuals. Disabled people are individuals. We have a sense of humour too. We can laugh at ourselves. Indeed, for some of us, laughing is what keeps us going. All I seek, personally, is the normal respect you would give anyone.*

The Times 11 June 2016 I wrote to Melanie ...to congratulate her on her Queen's Birthday Honour...

Fabulous news in the Queen's Birthday Honours. Simply perfect. A huge thank you from everyone out here for breaking those rarely spoken of taboos ... from catheters to wheelchairs.... Husbands and dogs ...and everything in between ...it really helps. Thank your awesome lady. I still giggle every time my 'Dave' lets himself 'stand for one minute' to cook supper in the microwave obeying the structions on the packet allow to stand for one minute taken too literally...

Extract2 from Times 11 June 2016: Motivational Brave Educational (MBE)

*MBE= **M**otivational for others in the same position, **B**rave as in those out there helping us, **E**ducational, giving us able bodied a poke in the eye to pay more attention to the needs of others.*

14. Bugoff Oneoff, Wed, 14 Sep 2016

'Get your life back…take a device-break' the newspapers extolled that week. We did……it's called Cornwall. Thank goodness Cornish broadband and mobile connectivity meant that away from the cottage, no-one could get me. Luxurious surfing helped disengage much. We had a brilliant time. Meanwhile, Dipstick and I saw each other nearly every week. Either inpatient or out, over the June July time. He suggested a supra-pubic catheter. That is, catheter through the abdomen. I'd had one before. He pronounced me a 'ONE OFF' not able to find an evidence base for someone like me. To my advantage the bladder has such little sensation that it cannot even feel the catheter. Dipstick did the procedure under general anaesthetic in London, on one of the hottest days and nights of the year. The hospital provided a fan. But whoop it was hot. A soggy cold wet towel on the plastic hospital mattress provided a sort of relief. However, good news. We were now Week 3 and amazingly it was easy. Bladder was calm. But there were issues over the 'wound' it had created a right old mess. GP and nurse professed they were not suprapubic aware, not wound aware, they suggested asking Dipstick. We better add that to the mandatory Health professional training. My blood pressure was too high, the gp changed those meds too. I messaged Dipstick. He replied eventually, a short sharp three words. Tried to get help from experts, wound care helpline, district nurses, FFS....got nowhere fast...everyone thought it was an indwelling, argghghghgh...you are such a one-off no-one seemed to know what to do, tried Dipstick again. No response. Tried Wingrave, no luck. I guess it was conference season. It is the equivalent of bugger off we are busy.... BUGOFF – ONEOFF, sort yourself out. Using my secret code (#anaphylactic!) I managed to request GP, Saint Pee, to ring me. He was brilliant and tried hard. I managed to get past 'Rottweiler-on-call' without a murmur...It worked. He rang. HURRAH. BP stuff causing massive migraines he tried changing tack on medications, creams for wound, drugs for wound, dressings.

15. BLADDER BUDDY, SAT, 24 SEP 2016

I'd had weird dreams that week. Must have been the aftereffects of Massive Migraines (MM). The journal entry this day was:

I dreamt I went to be 'reprogrammed' in London. On my way met an Irish engineer who had invented running shorts which support pelvic floors for ladies. I dreamt I wore them to Pilates and managed to do the splits (sort of) wearing them, which went on twitter I panicked that the suprapubic was leaking again. In fact, the warm cosy damp feeling was my mobile phone overheating with fruit gums stuck to it. what else did I dream? I dreamt I went back to this hospital for a third time and found to my considerable delight the Wi-Fi recognised me straight away as a frequent visitor. That Jerome was there and calmed my nerves about leaking catheters by explaining the Bladder Buddy technique...bin bag over the head *(you tube http://youtu.be/IdUMy9HzdWo)*[27] But that made me laugh much (again) I had to check for leaks and grab my empty water bottle just in case. Later, our neighbour's daughters regaled me with stories of music festivals and 'she-wees' to avoid the horrible toilets. Mixed up in all this nonsense I bumped into Elm on the train home. She wondered if I would be a volunteer for her brides' fair event. 'Me?' I yelled incredulously for all

---

[27] Bladder Buddy technique...bin bag over the head (you tube http://youtu.be/IdUMy9HzdWo).

the train to hear. 'Well,', she said 'we are doing alternative wedding ideas, gay, transgender, older ladies, wider ladies....' ohhhhhh of course...not sure which category she had in mind. 'How about I demonstrate wedding dresses for ladies with catheters' I said. 'Bladder-buddy and she-wee at the ready'. We howled with laughter to the dismay of the very important looking busy commuters tapping away on their laptops. One of whom, started praying, next to me.... for emergency deployment of his invisibility cloak or for my soul? Lost cause. Then, just to add to the madness I find myself guiding my daughter H to a bridal wear shop. I'm on a train (again). H is in her hometown. I get her to stop for a drink on the way using my google app map doodah. She gets to try on the dresses I have already rung ahead to be organised. She sends me photos. I choose. She agrees. I pay. She smiles. That trainload of passenger's grin at this bizarre exchange. Not least her giggle 'well if I cannot find something, I like I will just go naked!' There is only one thing more I can add: None of this was a dream.

It all happened that week.

Sun, 06 Nov 2016 Prostate or Prostrate?

This is what I wrote in the blog:

.... I've been here in the waiting room for 3 hours now....

Bloody chaos but I really could not be arsed to care. The banter in the waiting room was funny...a poor gentleman on my right was very worried that it was always like this.

'It's my first time'. He spoke.

'I'm rather nervous that Dr Dip is in a bit of a state'.

'Don't worry'. I counselled.

'It's always like this. But he's really very good.'

The nice man wandered over to my seat and he whispered to me.... 'We ARE talking about the same doctor, are we...?' Is this normal for him,...its all a bit chaotic'? Do I do my PSA[28] here?

Summoning all my mentoring skills I chatted him into going to talk to the secretary for the missing information. He did. She sorted it. He wandered off. With a wink to me! Another patient was sitting there too. She was younger than the rest of us, giggling away. It was her birthday. We were all wishing her well. Oh well that killed another hour. The bloody pomegranate china display thing was beginning to get on my nerves. It's meant to depict a bladder. I think. I started to plan how I could accidentally push it out the window.

---

[28] PSA is a blood test for prostate cancer.

16. Trolley Dolly, Sat, 12 Nov 2016 another hospital stays

I was back in hospital and feeling terrible, the last iv intravenous (IV) drip of the day was going in. But late...the drugs trolley had capsized in the corridor outside, earlier, it had been a while before nurses had restored order. I had begun to look at hospital life like one flew over the cuckoo's nest.[29] New patients arrived relatively sane and ended up institutionalised stark raving bonkers. Dipstick kept telling me it or I, was hopeless I'm 'colonised', whatever that meant. To his credit he did not bat an eyelid when I petulantly declared 'so it's all my fault then'

---

[29] Kesey, K. (1976). One Flew Over The Cuckoo's Nest (1962). One Flew Over the Cuckoo's nest the story which is drama and comedy of patients in a psychiatric ward, one of whom is not needing psychiatric help. In the film starring Jack Nicholson, his character encourages the other inmates to rebel against the institutionalisation.

17. Absolute Dogs Bollocks, Sat, 03 Dec 2016

Extract from The Times 2nd December 2016 Spinal Column by Melanie Reid: Melanie and I have written to each other over the last few years. She is tetraplegic after breaking her neck and back in a riding accident in April 2010 in the paper today she wrote:

.... where we are the champions, the bizzo, the absolute dog's b******s, is in the expression of gratitude. We spend our entire bloody lives thanking people for helping us. In fact, I would say I have a master's degree in supplication and gratitude: read these practised lips – they say ten dozen can I/would you/please pass me/thank yous every single day. Because sometimes, you know, that is all we have inside left to give. Humdrum words. And sincerity. A Master's degree in the absolute dogs b*******.

Oh, my days this resonated. There I was lying in hospital.

THANKYOU I said as the nurse yanked out the SPC (Supra Pubic Catheter).

THANKYOU for answering the call bell.

THANKYOUUUUUUUUU …. please could I,

Excuse me…

SORRY, THANKYOU, THANKYOU

…. gratitude argh. As for the bloody ceiling. I had suggested a starry glow star thing on the ceiling would be a considerable improvement…. tut … forgetting myself. I should say THANKYOU for putting the bed flat. All I can do is scrabble about like an upside-down tortoise! THANKYOU!

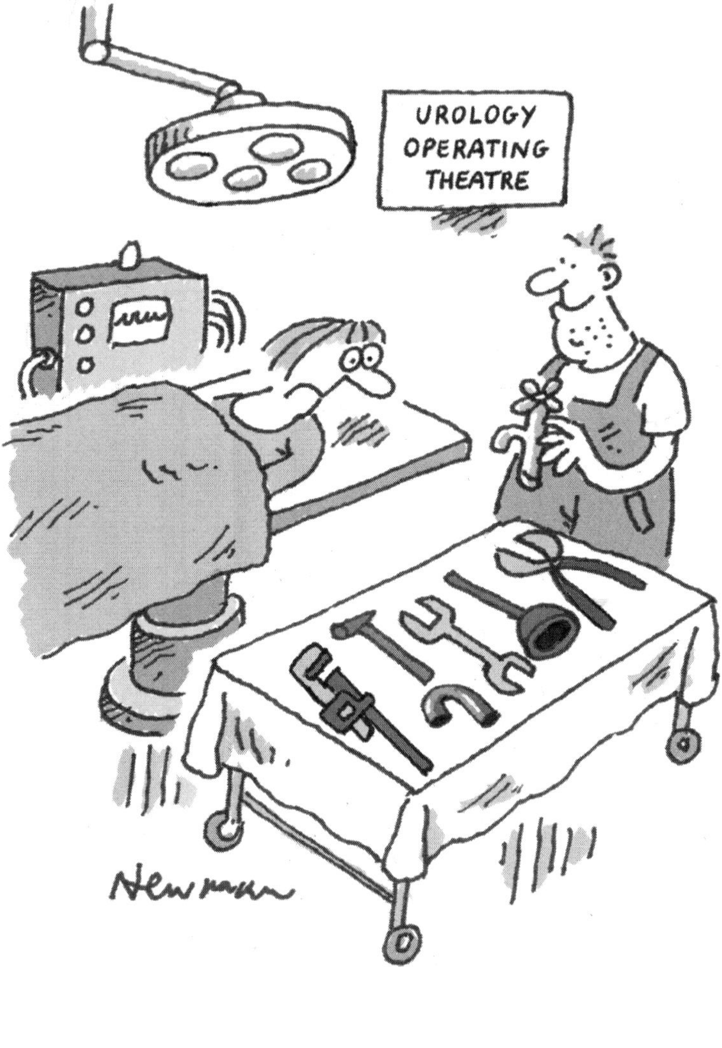
UROLOGY
OPERATING
THEATRE

18. Why are you Here, Mon, 30 Nov

This Monday was a routine check-up with the renal team who removed kidney 1.

Having been to this clinic a few times. Usually, it is easy. This time:

Consultant called me in. *'Why are you here?'*

I've read my screen I cannot understand why you have an appointment.

Fighting down the urge to scream and run I calmly explained.

1. Your team removed my kidney.
2. I've been coming for check-up of renal function and blood pressure ever since.
3. The last time I was here the consultant wrote copious notes and felt it important to have 6 monthly appointments.
4. The story started in 2009…. I produced my own notes, drugs list, allergy list and he feverishly wrote it up. His sweaty shirt was hanging out, hot sweaty tired unshaven…goodness knows what emergencies he'd had to handle …then me his last patient of the day.

19. Squashed bananas, Sat, 10 Dec 2016

Somewhere or other I had lost November and now gradually the dawning realisation that we were halfway through Advent. When did that happen? Truth to tell I had shivered and shuddered through infection 1 and infection 2. I had been in hospital a fair bit. I had seen a lot of Three Men in A Boat i.e., the surgeons who looked after me. Not forgetting Uncle Montmerency. Suprapubic was taken out. IV antibiotics had been blasted. Now we were trying a bit of immune boost. And hope. As Jerome might say: *'Hoping is always good'*.

The hospital team had been brilliant. I even had a visit from the head chef for feedback.

'Toast' I said. 'Too floppy' I said. 'How about a toast rack, dry it out a bit?' Bloody hell he did it too!

20. Mice and men, Fri, 16 Dec 2016

I was sitting in a luggage rack …again. London bound train. No seats. Luggage rack had free Wi-Fi because it' was next to first-class. Now that is always -a -positive The First class was full of important men tapping laptops shouting into phones…oh to be one of the alpha men! I was on route to a Board meeting at NH England, EICC. The day before I had been to London to see Dipstick for a check-up. He had clearly been on a 'be-nice-to-patients' course. He smiled! Shook my hand!?? Was EARLY.

Went through options.

Drew nice diagrams.

He was GREAT. I mentioned Montmorency's data. A European project. Trial of new stuff. Cost £7k a week! But only on mice so far.

Dipstick replied: 'but you are not a mouse'. Well at least that is clear. I found myself telling him how I had snuck a mouse in a biscuit tin on a plane to Geneva. (I was 10 and going to see my parents. – Even got mention on radio 4). Dipstick just stared at me… ('eye-contact-course') shook his head and got rid of me as fast as he could. Receptionist said he had had a few cancellations!! I will tell the full mouse story another day….

21. CAKES AT CHRISTMAS LONG LIVE THE NHS

Thu, 12 Jan 2017 It's official. NHS is awesome. As Patsy said…long live the NHS we love you. Allergy clinic was on the Friday in the airport style high rise building down the Euston Road … whatever it was they tried, I had a horrible reaction by the time I had got home …She emailed me through the night as the reaction raged,

My foot had swollen like a balloon, the pain level hit 10+ ……and the antidotes worked to keep me out of and…

We did it somehow. Jerome also pitched in on Saturday with antibiotic advice….and Mr Hunt says we do not have a 24/7 service. Then on Wednesday back for another Allergy challenge day. Amazing rabbit warren of a hospital outpost. In fact, this the very hospital I spent many hours in, when my father had his brain tumour operation here. 1985. My mother was so squeamish, I parked her in the pub next door.

Dr Allergy greeted me like a long-lost friend…. We talked, we planned, we researched. We looked through all the msu results I had. We worked it out together…. we needed Uncle Montmerency…like NOW. She got the switchboard to bleep him. Phew. He answered. They talked for ages. Hatched a plan. Back home once more, hoping the night would be alright, I was due back the day after.

Messages

Morning J Hope you are feeling Ok Did you see the programme about St Marys? Well, about the NHS really. Or about the extraordinary solidarity between clinicians, organisers and their patients fighting against the lack of supply... Truly extraordinary – but just like it is, every day. Jerome

22. Patients, virtue and patience, Mon, 27 Feb 2017

I have always thought the use of 'lost my kidney' a bit odd. Like I left my kidney somewhere and now cannot remember where. Now if it were my keys. That is another story. Kidney Anniversary was in fact Wednesday. It was 29th Feb 2012 leap year. Recipient and I ... We exchange letters and cards, he was doing well, in fact he had changed from a 'nearly dead' to a 'nearly wed'. My bladder infections raged on. Antibiotics? I kept bunging in. I could not be arsed to appeal for help.... I did not want the hassle for the men in the boat.

How on earth do these doctors do it? 24/7 day after day. Night after night. I hope most patients are appreciative and not as petulant as me! Word on the street, we have many retired doctors living near us, GPs get paid more than surgeons. They work 5 days a week. Extra for nights and weekends. Err...hang on a minute. That does not seem quite right. What business model would let that through?

Life in NHS Hospital-land is tougher, more stressed than anything. There was I thinking teaching was tough and stressy. I have started a book my nephew recommended to me... am slowly taking it in. It's called the' Innovator's Prescription' by Christensen[30], based really

---

[30] Christensen, C. M., Grossman, J. H., & Hwang, J. (2009). The innovator's prescription. A disruptive Solution for.

on the USA but some brain challenging ideas. The bit I was particularly interested in is 'Disruptive Solutions for the care of Chronic Disease'. What I was beginning to appreciate is that the NHS was built to optimise management of acute crises or episodes. Diagnose the chronic disease, evaluate its progression and sort ensuing complications. Check. But, what about monitor, encourage adherence to prescribed therapy. Does anyone have the time? The capacity? To give care during the adherence stage.

23. Pacing, Gin and Caffeine, Wed, 01 Mar 2017

On Wed, 1 Mar 2017 at 05:30, after 1000 phone calls, letters, and emails I had to turn up as instructed at the pain clinic in London… I'd had many letters cancelling/changing and I was in a right muddle. Having missed the last one as I was ill in hospital it turned out I was booked for a group follow up session. 11.00 to 15.00. I thought it was an appointment with the rep to sort reprogramming on my spinal implant Nevro[31] reset. I explained (truthfully) I had to get home for a meeting and no way could I stay till 3:00. Eventually the session started. Some sad stories as each person introduced themselves. I tried to be sensible and showed I could move by standing up every now and again, pacing around wiggling. (So that's what PACING was?) They asked what strategies we used to cope with the frustrations of breakthrough pain etc. I said: my best strategy was pouring a gin! And go for an open-air swim. It did not go well.

---

[31] Nevro High Frequency Spinal implant.

24. What a laugh, Wed, 12 Apr 2017

I had an appointment with Dipstick that day because my Sacral Nerve Implant (SNS) which helps my bladder to work, seemed not to be working. Of course, he was running late. But he got my name right. I tried to skate over the mysterious big wave wipe out which occurred last week in Cornwall. I said I was swimming. True. I said I 'might' have banged my back. True. Maybe possibly. I had knocked my SNS. Err. I explained I had to turn it off as it seemed to be stimulating my toes and shoulder not my bladder! Odd that? EEK... He stared at me. Asked to see the (considerable) bruising. 'I don't understand how you did that'. He said.

Swimming, body boarding, waves, Cornwall....I could not run any more but swimming, I could do. Sea or lake. With a wet suit. When the water was too effing cold any pain dissolved. The odd leaking bladder just kept some warmth.... He actually laughed ...' I'm not sure who is the bigger kid you or me 'So now as I wrote my blog I was waiting for a scan, I would get the implant re-checked out the following week with the rep from the implant company and we kind of devised a plan, parting as friends, for once.

25. Piddles make puddles, Sun, 23 Apr 2017

Bladder news was bonkers. Much bonkers. In short: I had now had a non-stop infection since oh February. To be clear. That meant pain, headaches, back ache, smelly pee and spasms. Some days were better than others. Antibiotics were changed every so often. But each time I stopped the vomit-making high doses and moved onto the next antibiotic and hoped. Each week I sent an 'msu'. I.E., mid-stream urine sample, multi antibacterial clean sample. That was then sent to the 'lab' with a 'form'. I could have done that via my GP. He and I had devised a way of getting past the Rottweilers on his reception and the gatekeepers at the nurses' station. The reason for our devious plan, was that sample could be stopped at any moment by those very important receptionists and they had the 'POWER' to make sure that the test tube, was not sent to the 'lab'. The reception only allows one 'test tube' per person. Woe betides you if you lost it or, dropped it and then, GOD forbid, put your pee in an old JAM JAR. The nurses had the task of dip sticking the pee. That allowed them to reject any that did not register an infection. It also allowed for cross-contamination, false negatives, false positives and effing stupid effing false results. Now bear with me here. The 'lab', if the pee ever gets there, tests the msu. The results are generated. It takes a 48-hour culture growing slide to find the sensitivities and resistances to antibiotics. It did take a bit longer, if a particularly resistant bugger was found.

That lab report went to the GP. The GP scribbled on it. After a week, as instructed, the patient is instructed to ring for the result. If there was no growth of bacteria, the Rottweiler could say: 'Result normal no further action'. If (as was nearly always the case for me) the culture has grown a bug, Rottweiler would say 'you must speak to a doctor'. Then there was the inordinately antediluvian procedure to ask for an appointment with a usual doctor, (unlikely for 6 weeks) or a phone consultation (usually 1 week hence), or an appointment or phone call with ANY doctor (usually 48 hours) This all takes time of course and the infection symptoms just got worse and worse. I am lucky enough to see some London consultants too. Of these, Jerome, devised an excellent scheme where I had many pre signed 'forms' 'pots' and 'special plastic bags' - Thus armed I could catheter cleanly into pot, much easier than the GP bloody test-tube. Pot went to lab. If I was not in London, faithful Daniel drives the sample to work in North London. A taxi then takes it to the 'lab'. A cost implication which makes me hesitate every time as the lab and taxi cost meso much. BUT. When desperate (rather often of late) I got the result via Jerome, his phone, and my iPad, within 48 hours. I was able to get onto the right antibiotic and stand a fighting chance of beating the buggers. This could sometimes really really go tits up though.

Dipstick did not seem to be able to use his phone to receive the results. In fact, I felt he had a specific device on his phone that deleted all patient details, calls, texts, emails, and messages about patients. Not that I blamed him for trying to protect himself. It was just that every time I saw him, he insisted: *you know how to get hold of me.* NO, I DO NOT you are effing nightmare man. I have challenged him He really did insist that I could ring or text ANY TIME. FFFFFFRRRRRRRRRRR

I rang his office for the results. Very nice ladies said he had the result, and he would sort it.

He did not.

I texted him.

He did reply!

'Script sent' whatever the f that meant. Rang his poor office again. Turned out he had cleverly got them to organise a prescription. For the stuff I am ALLERGIC to.

I texted him.

He did not reply.

His office tried again.

Just send me the results I pleaded.

That was all I needed just the bloody results, please.

Eventually 8 days after the test they emailed the results.

In parallel I rang the GP for his results. Usual 'make an appointment next year' response. Health Economics I have been learning at NICE guidelines it, revolves around Quality-of-Life calculations. Opportunity costs and improved patient outcomes. How many piddles make a puddle?

From Jerome:

Email from Jerome to Jacq:

I will provide a brief analysis and then offer advice.

An MSU[32] is a sample of urine, otherwise it would be a pee.

If you produce a sample, then it must be analysed.

If it was not analysed, it cannot be a sample.

It was just some urine in a pot.

So, as you see, to have produced an MSU, which was a sample, it should go to a laboratory for tests.

The laboratory was based at xxx.

You could take the sample to the laboratory.

Alternatively, we have a courier service, which acts to take samples of urine (which was to say MSUs, produced by patients, which we want to have analysed) to the laboratory.

So, it was now clear that, whether you bring the sample to us, or take it to 'lab', it will end up at lab, and be analysed.

Surgeon Dipstick does not consult at the 'Lab', nor in fact does the Laboratory provide a consultation service. Indeed, as we have established, it does its best work analysing samples, such as MSUs, that have been produced by patients and end up at Lab either directly or indirectly as discussed in paragraph 2.

Accordingly, if we are to assume that when Dipstick suggested he see you for a few moments, he meant a brief consultation, it would seem logical that he meant where he consults as opposed to the 'lab' where he does not

---

[32] MSU Mid-Stream Urine;

Extrapolating the facts and suppositions into a conclusion, Dipstick will be at his clinic and can consult with you there, and your MSU sample can be sent from there to 'lab' for analysis. See Dipstick there) have our team send the sample to the 'lab' the result will come to us.

Too many of us (Drs) don't see it sufficiently from the patient's perspective. It was a salutary read.

I will see you at or around 1530. Not sure what my diary looks like but will certainly find 5 mins from somewhere to have a real-life chat.

For the benefit of my medical clear English campaign, and for both of our personal convenience, this will be best achieved at my surgery.

I can fill-form if form-unfound.

It was good that you are the patient voice for NHS (start small, work up)

Was the blog going to be a book? I'd be delighted to write a foreword. Or was it a preface? I got a B in English.

Bw

Messages from friends:

It was awful. I can hardly believe it you are such a victim of such a terrible system. Currently. It was too wearying for words, and you must be at the end of your tether... how can 'they' be so inefficient. It was terrible, terrible, terrible. If you saw the highest authority in the urologist land, do you think it would make things better? You see. To know better than any of the so-called specialists what should be done, but why the delays, and all the time your infections are thriving, and the cocktail of antibiotics cannot be good for you. Don't give up, don't give up.

Patsy wrote too:

I'm jumping up and down with frustration and anger on your behalf and just wished you lived in my area because I'm sure you would receive excellent treatment here. Anyhow it's time you came to see me for some TLC not to mention a delicious gin I picked up recently. I can't call you because I have no voice now, but I do have a sore throat and chest infection. We lose some, we gain some! All love Patsy

26. Hippo, Cock and Bull Story, Fri, 19 May 2017

I had made a hasty decision in a fit of energy and healthfulness…well all 24 hours of it…to visit my brother in Toronto with a subplot…to meet my youngest son, little 6'6", BFG, returning from his travels. Well, I went. UTI threatening…bunged in every bloody thing I could think of to fly across the Atlantic. Poured in the …. water…well a little champagne too…just a little. Medicinal. Fabulous brother and his fabulous Canadian wife met me. Waited on me hand and foot. Introduced the 'whacky-but-nice' neighbours. We all went to meet BFG, as he staggered off his flight. Whoop.exciting. many adventures to be related. Many hairy faced photos, blonde hair and sheer happiness. Brilliant. Vicariously brilliant. Doctors? Aha…well, I did find had felt bit crap in Toronto. I tried to pretend it was jet lag. I took some other antibiotics, I happened to have on me! I woke at night in a lather of coughing wheezing and fever…my wonderful sister-in-law happens to have a nurse daughter who manages the one and ONLY private clinic in Toronto. Lucky me. Appointment fixed. Seen by the ever-formal white coated Dr Seuss . . . Quick check-up. Quick diagnosis. Radiology lady. Poor lady turned a whiter shade of pale when she read my x-rays…I had forgotten to tell her about my metal implants. I am so so sorry I wheezed. I am bionic. I should have told you. OOPs…., bronchitis and pneumonia and asthma…and pharmacy…and more antibiotics, steroids, puffers…you name it I had it. Bloody brilliant and back in time to be wined and dined. Pizza oven outside to the fore. BFG and my brother and his wife sorted everything.

Dr Seuss looked like Robin Williams, in his film, Patch Adams, he had been careful to explain I could be seen at the 'Public' hospital but that I would have to pay by credit card up front. Not a lot different from his clinic. I stayed. He did make me promise to go to the EmergencyDepartment (ED) of Public Hospital, if any worse or no better. But politely reminded me of the charges once more. Interesting. Bet we don't insist on credit cards here. But then what happens if you are ill cannot pay and maybe won't pay…mm. free at the point of delivery? I got back to the UK. Full of antibiotics, the good thing was that my bladder seemed to like that massive cocktail. Next was a follow up appointment with Montmorency. He suggested various bladder potions. He also unofficially recommended vodka, steroid inhalers, codeine, antihistamine… and 3 days sleep for the cough!

Meanwhile my mother-in-law seemed unwell. I suggested the carers get her to the GP. Which they did. But not a lot happened. Thinking through all that they told me, I suggested perhaps a bladder infection might be the cause of fever, confusion and lethargy. Bugger me, I was right, and she ended up in hospital. My skills are becoming honed.

Messages

Bloody hell. Really?? There is me thinking you had a restful holiday in Canada. Appreciate it was not the sort of story you can reel off in five minutes but am sorry to hear all that -

.... Wow Jacq, I did not realise as usual that you had been through much again.... You always keep quiet about how many doses of millions of drugs you are on to keep you smiling and the life and soul of the Yellow Cardies – take care keep getting better (over and over again) as the next dose of whatever bug was thrown at you.... This made me laugh!

...Good and not good to hear all this. Hope you are back safely. Health services in Canada sound a lot better than here. And imagine you fixing your mother-in-law by remote control diagnosis and telling them what to do. Hope you are ok.

27. Prosecco, Sat, 03 Jun 2017

It had been another weird week. After seeing Dipstick, the previous week, the pulsing frequency of the bladder implant known as SNS reached unbelievable levels. Hot pain radiating down hip and right leg...even twitching toes. I had to turn the whole thing down gradually and then off. The positive of that was that it proved an excellent distraction to the ever-growing bug situation. By the end of the long bank holiday weekend swallowing paracetamol downing copious litres of water and shivering with cold despite the 27' outside, tried to act normal, got odd looks as I wore my fleece outside but got away with it somehow. Tuesday dawned bright and warm. Early train to London was boarded and I went to see Wingrave. Cleverly I had worked out how to get the rep for the bladder implant (SNS) to turn up at his clinic, having failed spectacularly to get her to Dipstick's the previous week. I made it on time having sat on the luggage rack of the early train! Rep turned up soon after me. Saw the big man himself. He was on dapper form full of jokes and smiles. Wrote his inky update on medical bits whilst the rep fiddled with the SNS paddles. That's bionic for you. What was that film ...Jason Bourne? Where he has the secret code embedded in his hip. Or CIA chip in his arm. Err maybe that was another film. Seemingly poor old Dipstick had managed last week to create a spectacular short circuit implosion. She reset it. I thanked her. Wingrave agreed to my suggestions: MSU I said, needed.

Antibiotics. I spoke. Prescription for. OK. He spoke. And I escaped…well nearly. There was some confusion about where the 'msu' forms and pots and toilets. For that were to be found. An hour later having been up and down the stairs 4 times, I had produced said 'sample'. Feeling a bit hot and clammy…. I tried to make the great escape. Made it to within 5 metres of the exit door but …next thing I knew the Wingrave and lots of nurses were flapping around. Suggesting ambulances to and or admission to his hospital there. I had had a bit of a collapse down at the entrance door, bugger. Decisions made I was wheeled off to a room. Bed, DUVET!! And being looked after by possibly the nicest kindest on call doctors and nurses you can imagine. Some knew me of old and greeted me with such sympathy I nearly cried. Freezing cold but sweating, pain like everywhere, I was made comfortable assured I would 'soon be home' and slept the rest of the day away. Massive antibiotic gentamicin was injected quickly into muscle in my leg…. Drips up. Painkillers in. News travelled fast. Bestest of visitors arrived with prosecco which they drank (I could not face that), Wingrave came in next day. All jollies. Demanding my blood test results, urine culture and diagnosis. I had to weakly admit to him I simply had none of the information he required perhaps the ward staff would help him, after all he was the surgeon in charge! So, he suggested I go home?!! I told him I thought some more gent would be good. He agreed. I suggested a course of antibiotics might be good. He agreed. 4 seconds later he was gone...with wonderful, worried staff rushing in to find he'd disappeared in a puff of...? that's we did. Home I went. Nurses nervously telling me to come straight back at the slightest thing. Daniel sorted chocolate for staff, cab and train for us. (We left (empty) prosecco bottle ...in the luggage rack!) Friday, I persuaded the hospital to release my various results. They ended up on the desk of Jerome's secretary. The hospital could only post not email. They could however fax? Who the hell has a fax anymore? I had scrambled in my bag for a fax number. The first I found, was the Urology centre where Jerome was based. Anyhow, results I now had, thanks to secretary of Jerome. Now what?

28. Marbles ... lost my, Sat, 10 Jun 2017

Massive thankyou to Melanie Reid who highlights the inexorable cycle of urinary tract infections., in Times spinal column. I had drafted a letter... *Dear Mel, I have just read your article in today's paper.*

Marbles? I lost mine years ago...you are utterly brilliant at putting into words this most exhausting cycle of uti episodes. I LOVE D mannose. Do not know what it does and frankly do not care! I'll try the garlic you describe. Gin was good. Fizz better. Does bugger all for the bladder but induces a booster to bran. Dr Vodka would agree, I'm sure. Allergy J has a nurse who prescribes Brazilian rum. But I digress... there's another potion called Uromune. I got some via German Pharmacy. It didn't seem to help. However, I've found out there's a new version.

A certain Dr FOLEY (can you believe the surname!!!) The effing FOLEY catheter was part of the problem! Sorry, where was I? Oh yes. Dr Foley was running a trial. BUT also, he was able to sell the stuff. No way am I going on a trial. Just my luck I'd get the frigging smarties placebo which would give me a massive migraine. There's not a proper evidence base. They have used it a lot in Spain with good results. The results favour the vaccine as an effective strategy for recurrent UTIs. However, they do not 'do' the evidence quite like in UK. Mananya...

Anyhow.... The huge joke was it's meant to be started when the patient was NOT on antibiotics and with a clear msu culture. That rules me out! Best of marbles to you me x

PS My irascible late father-in-law used to wander about looking for his pipe. Muttering 'I've lost my…I've lost my…I've lost my ….' Our youngest, Little G, or BFG as he's now known interjected… "Marbles?" Only BFG could get away with that!

29. BONKERS, SUN, 02 JUL 2017

To quote Jerome, this week had been utterly *bonkers*. I was guessing he had dissolved into a cocktail of bonkers for at least the previous 6 months, so quiet had he been. For now, here was a flavour... Wednesday: I was up at crack of dawn. Packed. Power dressed. Well, work shirt and jacket type power! Dog done. Early train (was sitting in the luggage rack as usual). Made it after a crazy tube situation to ever serious guideline meeting in the mall. On my very best behaviour, no jokes, serious face. Halfway through the first presentation I looked down at my shirt...it was inside out! Much for the power dress thing! OMG. Waited for the coffee interval, casual as I could, slipped away to the toilets for a tidy up! ...long day there, then over to an anonymous hotel somewhere in Regents Park for a power nap and change of clothes. (The right way around). Thank goodness I set 3 alarms, struggled to wake up and sort myself out... I was the pre-dinner speaker at a Continence Live event. The guests were clinicians from UK. I did tell them a few serious bits. Then I moved onto the story of falling into the Triathlon Lake. In fact, I did a whole simulation. I asked one of the Directors to assist me as I removed a bunch of flowers from a large glass vase. It was full of water, part of hotel decor. My assistant then had to dunk a continence pad into the vase. At the same time, I distributed a few pads on sundry tables, and asked guests to slowly pour water over the pads. Whilst all this was happening, I told my story of the rescue boat taking me back to the athlete's podium and my attempts to regain access to our room. At the very end of the story, I asked all the volunteers to hold up the pads (or take out of the vase). This I explained to loud giggles was exactly like the incident in the lake. It looked and felt like a blooming lifeboat between my frigging legs. I got many laughs! The poor waiters looked distinctly nervous. Serious point. Rationing pads does not make any sense. 3 pads a day was not enough. You cannot expect for example, a leaking gentleman newly discharged after prostatectomy, to sit in a soggy, wet, jelly, life-raft type pads all day... That was simply unfair. Quality of life, dignity, confidence, and the rest.

We went off to Cornwall after that, for a relaxing holiday ...but

Of course, I had a UTI which just would not budge whatever I threw at it. I had an appointment with Dipstick for check-up. Not much he could suggest. But sent another msu.

Someone rang saying Dipstick wanted to send a prescription. Great. But the office didn't know my chemist. That was CRAP. I've had the same scary chemist since this whole effing nightmare started in 2009 and they know it. I calmly gave the name etc. I was polite HONEST. 5:00 pm phone rings again. We have rung the chemist and they don't have the stuff. Office now closed. That is that then. I do not even know what the 'stuff' was. Maybe Dipstick could tell me. Maybe I have it already.

Maybe my GP will help. But why would that matter. Who bloody cares? Bladder and kidney are doing wonderfully crystalline boomerang firework impressions.

Messages:

I can hardly believe the medical nightmare goes on. And on. And on. Why can-t they get their act together and behave like normal responsible folk. Do you think they are reading this? If they should be blushing, they should apologise, they should say, and mean, 'we will look after you from now onwards and stop being unnecessarily inefficient.' How difficult was it to do things properly, rather than badly? You are amazing to be laughing.

To complete the last episode chapter and verse on the prescription that never arrived. Having found I could get a phone signal, by hanging over fence post 5, on the main road. Rottweiler GP receptionist told me I was extremely irritating to have had a phone signal. I forbore from asking her if I should quickly rig up a new mobile mast base station. Rottweiler eventually found a fax-email-record of Dipstick's request. Her helpful comment was: As you know you must allow 3-4 days to process a prescription. My foul-mouthed expletives, I swear (!) I never used to bloody swear like I have in the last few weeks, got tangled in the mobile crackle as I tried to explain this was an urgent request from a London Consultant 10 days ago. I might as well have said it was written by my postman for all the difference it made to her. I did attempt a request to speak to a doctor. But quickly stopped as she pretended this was impossible less than two days ahead and I was thinking I'd have to sit in the road for hours days weeks hoping for a signal to pick up the unknown; caller id which signifies the GP private call which cannot be missed. Oh, hell this was all raps. In the background my dear friend and retired doctor, albeit paediatrician, was driving rage fuelled furiously between surgery and chemist. She was giving Rottweiler what for on my behalf. Eventually, goodness knows how, she got 3grams of this bloody stuff to me by express delivery. Now what?

30. Dragon Tattoo, Tue, 22 Aug 2017

I was in Sussex for a photo shoot. Staying with Patsy my 'living-with-cancer' friend. We've shared much over 25 years. Mainly monsoons of tears…of laughter… mind you carefully…both of us wary of our bladders. Oh, by the way we now have even shared our decrepit left eye issues…. of course, when I arrived, we quickly ran through agenda before going indoors to meet the 'cameras'.

Her Effing Cancer was back, big time…. latest scan and hospital appointment last week. Plans to be made this week. Options. Or stop. TBA. We swore very very loudly, badly, outside, and then decided to open some fizz…laughing crazily as we walked to the front door.

Agenda item 2: Follow up to Rottweiler receptionist story. NO. That stupid idea did not work. Yes, the uti was back. Antibiotics which? Dunno? Don't care. I had lost all confidence in the London doctors. END OF…. SO… Ready…. for the photo shoot, it really deserved a whole story of its own. For now, let's just say the photographer was a wonderful sensitive charming young lady from Sweden. She had been assigned the brief for a large organisation to provide photos of 'hygiene' / 'health'. She had met and photographed many patients. Perhaps we two would have been the quirkiest. We laughed, talked, and posed and laughed even more for 24 hours. We practiced our Swedish phrases. My best attempt was

Steig Larsson. Really ... maybe I was a bit tired! The 'Bridge' didn't translate well! Calendar girls it was not. Decorum preserved but I certainly did not need my vast hold-all alternative outfits I had rather naïvely packed. You should have heard us laugh about that. Mind you, I personally was most relieved that the post-man arrived **after** the coffee break.

That week continued in the style of a roller coaster. I was missing the wonderful Pippi Longstocking photo shoot already. My amazing cool Patsy had shown me her cancer decision -tree -flowchart so I sent her a message: Nolite Te bastardes carborundorum—I had read that in a book. Don't let the buggers get you down.

31. Shaggy Dog, Mon, 11 Sep 2017

Here I was again. The screaming hilarious laugh a minute Health Show. Urodynamic. God I how I hated bloody urodynamics, but it was at a different place. Trying to avoid the awfulness of the past, fifty shades of nightmare. It was all worth it. Lucky me to have a precious appointment fast. It was 4 months ago it was booked. Speedy, eh? Having kept bladder full as instructed. Always a bit of a nightmare in case it spontaneously erupts en route. After 5 phone calls and 3 texts all reminding me of my appointment, I had great hopes of organisational greatness.

I had even had a phone call that morning to check I was coming. Wow. Even got a phone call as I boarded my expensive train down. Got a seat! It was all going well. I was asked on this last call to please get there early as they were running ahead of time. Early? Wow. Impressive. Keep bladder full was the instruction. OK I'll get there as fast as the train takes me. I had said. I hoped bladder held out and not spontaneously erupt. I arrived. Receptionist could never be called 'Rottweiler' more of a podgy unsmiling shaggy dog ... a .... shaggy sheepdog pushing patients about looking disinterested. He was having a lovely listen to something through his earphones. Tapping away to the 'beats. I managed to get his attention. He took my letter. Thrust a form at me. I filled that in... ALLERGIC to contrast? Yes. Kidney issues? Yes wash.......Etc. etc... Down to pregnant? NO! He was delighted and even smiled when I gave it back. Hah you haven't filled in your name. He chortled. Bet that gets him smiling every time. He went back to his beats, and I wandered about till I encountered a poor bloke sitting looking vulnerable in his 'gaping gown' not a stitch on other than that. Must be the right place I mumbled. He was too embarrassed to reply. Seconds later an official looking person hoiked him into a room called 'imaging'. Poor bloke getting his giblets zapped in his gaping-gown. FFS wasn't there a better frigging gown invented yet? I paced around a bit. Eventually a nice lady in blue came along. If I said. Sheepishly. You'd have guessed this was going to be the punchline. She said my name. She said she'd rung earlier to ask me to hurry there. YES. Bad news.... THE effing bloody machine had broken down in the relatively short time since we had spoken. Now what happens I asked meekly wondering if this could really be true. Maybe they just needed to go home early? You will 'get a letter' said. I turned tail. Left my stupid bladder diary stuff on the shaggy man's desk. He was still tuning in to his music. I tried to find the toilets to empty the 'kept full bladder'. But I dove for cover when I saw a consultant I know. Hid myself behind a pillar and avoided him. One of the men-in-the-boat. Didn't feel I could speak other than screaming. Back on to the train. Frrrrrrrrrrrrrrrrrrrrrr...No seats...luggage rack again.... screeeeeaaammmmmmm

32. Royal College of Testicles, Fri, 15 Sep 2017

Patsy and I saw a preview of our Pippi Longstocking photos. We were sworn to secrecy for fear Hello magazine got wind of it. As if. But we giggled. I think and hope a good distraction as her chemo kicked in once more. Frrrrrigitt. In answer to some emails about Urodynamic. Just to explain that it's a test to check out pressures (or lack of) in Bladder. Jerome was the only one who ever explained it well. He explained the maths understood. It's a wire up the bum. A wire and catheter in the bladder. X ray imaging. Bladder filled with saline. As it fills patient was asked to say when there was any sensation to pee. Gets to a point where they tip the X-ray table upright (with you on it, clinging for dear life) and patient then asked to pee. Yes, they do pretend to leave you some privacy. But only from behind a stupid screen. FFS. it is kind of intimate personal stuff. It is a bit pointless for someone like me as the pee won't pee! One reason I don't like it was the last time I had a male nurse and a male consultant doing the test. Now, I have no objection to male doctors or nurses at all. It's just that as I rarely feel any sensation of 'fullness', rarely able to pee with much success let alone when being tipped up …. Let alone when being stared at … kind of Fifty Shades of Grey … But it's not great. And no, it was not a nice test. Not sure why the patient reported symptoms are not believed. What does the test really change in terms of treatment? But hell, what does the patient know? She's only the patient. The Royal College of Obstetrics and Gyny has apparently only ever had two female presidents in its long history. A tweet I read this week suggests that if it were a Royal College of Testicles men would prefer that to be led by men. Just saying…

33. ON THE WRONG PLATFORM, SUN, 24 SEP 2017

Living with chronic conditions was a bit like travelling by train. To try to explain…. Whilst my parents named me the French long Jacqueline …they quickly realised that this was a mouthful and a half. So, thinking I could not spell. Referred to me as J.A.C.Q. to discuss of note. It has stuck to this day. I think they realise I can spell now. Certainly as 30% of my peers were named after Mrs Jackie Kennedy, I was mighty glad to assume a less obvious namesake. Perhaps it was in relation to my parents' favourite films… In the 50's a French actor, Jacques Tati. Jacques Tati made a series of films about the character Mon Oncle. A memorable clip was a train station platform. Incomprehensible announcements to waiting passengers … last minute trains arriving on wrong platforms with everyone trotting up the stairs over the bridge and onto the platform. …you get my drift? Having got stuck on a Sunday Service train for ages…in tunnel…having had to trot over to a last-minute change platform when I got on…spilt my coffee…got mopped up by lovely station man…I had a chance to reflect. Healthcare. It's one long change of platform after another. All valiant attempts to understand the commentary. Dashed in a moment. Looking confident in one place only to find I really needed to be in another. Lots of letters inviting me to appointments. Lots of letters cancelling those appointments. New letters inviting me to new appointments. Incomprehensible phone messages. Incomprehensible changes. Am I on the right plat-platform? To be continued…

34. BAPS, Wed, 27 Sep 2017

To continue Mon Oncle or Monsieur Hulot. That train station scene. Wrong platform, wrong train, and wrong time…place…! It's NHS week for me. Monday. (Eyes) Pre op assessment for a cataract, the left eye has seemingly deteriorated the only explanation seemed to be the various drugs and bugs I had been taking over the last years. Scans. Measures. Eyesight. The lady looking after me, explained that staff shortages were serious There had been a death amongst her clinic staff. A death and an itu case…staff in bits. That little piece of info made all the difference. 'Blimey how d' you cope with that on a Monday morning in a full clinic?' I asked. 'I just smile', she replied. We ended up best of friends. Me even extolling the virtues of my awesome spinal implant. She's got neck stuff to cope with. We laughed together. We agreed to update each other! Tuesday, check-up day for said spinal implant. Usually a good appointment. Rep and I get most of the programming sorted and leave the clinic team to tick the boxes. My appointment was 15:15. I was standing in the bloody nattering receptionist queue at 15:09. Eventually I get clocked in. A nurse arrived. 'Oh, we thought you weren't coming'. It was 15….27 he said But, but I said, I was in the building at 15.08 and waiting upstairs…. arg ghghghgh. Not a good start. I'd bloody broken world records to get there. A Rep from the implant company was there in the consulting room. At least I think it was. Never seen this one before. No name. Just the programming machine. Which she silently fiddled with. Mr Nurse asked his stupid questions. I answered without adjectives. I've found that to be quicker in the past.

Any problems? No

Any drugs? No thanks.

Any pain? The usual.

NB this WAS a pain clinic!

Goodness knows what his notes say! BAP? Bloody Annoying Patient. BAPS Bloody Annoying Patients. I did explain the need to combine the implant P1 and P2 to be P3. You see I've done this a while now. It's called SELF MANAGING. Mr Nurse looked surprised when I announced, 'right that's great I can go now'. His hand-written boring notes took a slide to the end. I did remember to ask. Please could he tell the chief pain team nurse that I was jolly grateful to receive 6 identical letters inviting me to her four -bloody -hour -group -therapy session. But please could I decline. You see, as I explained to him. I'd have to take another whole day off, AND I find it too depressing. The other patients hate the implants they've been given. They are sky high on morphine. When they are not crying, they are asleep. I can't help them. They can't help me. I LOVE my implant. Yes, it takes an hour to charge every day. Yes, it's awkward. But it WORKS. Let's thank the NHS for this expensive bit of kit. But as D says. We are meant to be ready at the drop of a hat any time, any day, cancel work for a precious appointment. For a precious procedure.

Put your life on hold. Woe betides you if you are late, or even a teeny bit just on time. The nurse with POWER will crazily moan at you. I sped back to my train. Just missed one by 30 seconds. The train crew obstinately locked the doors despite us passengers on the platform. POWER CRAZE. I got the next one and sped into my 'pretend-I'm-a teacher' meeting. Just as it ended! Eventually I got home. It was Tuesday and the rest of the week to come. A Mr Hulot scene that springs to mind. He's on holiday. He just carries on despite the chaos he causes! ……

Messages in:

Loved this, Jacq. Made me feel better about my melt down this morning over being forced to live like a student with some of the kids here… Hair in the plughole, damp washing everywhere, mashed potatoes all over the dishwasher.

35. NHS Hospital Wednesday, Wed, 27 Sep 2017

I could not let a day go by without an update from NHS land. The week of NHS-land continues.... I took Daughter 1 to her routine check-up. Only a few hours later and we staggered out with crashing headaches. Why are hospitals unbelievably hot? Why was everything on scruffy bits of paper? Why does NO-ONE introduce themselves? Give their name? Acknowledge the person WITH the patient does the doctor not look up while she was handwriting her copious boring illegible notes? Make eye contact. Do not assume the patient has a Scooby do what you are talking about. 'NAD' on a urine test. You have no idea that an otherwise intelligent person, in an anxious state, assumes that the nurse was somehow telling the Registrar some secret code. I know, you know, we all know…but in stress the patient brain goes very foggy. It all was ok just so slow and frustrating and hot. Poor clinicians working there. They must have crashing headaches too. One funny bit: A nurse came running out into the waiting room and asked the assembled crowd if anyone had seen a lady 'in a skirt'? We had great fun imagining what that might mean. An escapee from the examination room? A stripper? Maybe only a skirt and nothing else? We never did find out.

36. STOPCOCK, SUN, 08 OCT 2017

Short paragraph …tried not to use screens on account of my amazing new bionic eye…. For now, a story, that had made me laugh and laugh. My long-suffering family have been kind enough to ignore my myopic text messages and pretend it was predictive being predictive. However, during the week, I had to explain by text, a bit of a saga about water leaks, and I hasten to add, avoided the obvious bladder – leak innuendo. My text read: *'I had to tell them. To check the stopcock.'* My hilarious daughter 2, texted back: *'mums you are very funny.'* This evening when we spoke…she said she showed my text to her friends, and they all had a good laugh. *Fancy writing stopcock…what word were you trying to type?* She really really did not know that. Neither seemingly did her friends. Useless mother am I that I never taught her the rudiments of plumbing. The analogies with bladder are just too close, bet you there was some urological device which correlates…let's ask Jerome….I would plan the blog and would for now stop typing and laughing. PS bionic eye was ok and a story for another time. . . .

Messages:
- *Bionicle stopcock loved the Daily Stent, which made me laugh. It also reminded me of when I sent a pc to J on his Gap Year asking him how he was getting on in Bang Cock…*

37. ONE FLEW OVER THE CUCKOO'S NEST, FRI, 13 OCT 2017

I had tried not to annoy Dipstick or Jerome to source some antibiotics. Ended up filling poor Jerome's inbox yet a -bloody-gain. Cutting a long story short Dipstick had sent a script. But it was rejected by the chemist on account of it being *3 days' worth for a month*. Scary chemist didn't think that fitted any of his protocols. Jerome's response was brilliant. I hoped he did not mind me adding it here: *Sorry that Dipstick restricted it to 3 days. Bit overly optimistic that, given that you've only been off antibiotics for about 3 days this year… a triumph of hope over experience. But you've got to admire the optimism.bw J.*

With that chuntering on in the background I'd also run out of eye drops. The hospital gave me drops to take home. One bottle for two weeks. The other for four weeks. Steroid's antibiotics blah. Simple. Turns out the smaller 5ml bottle was for four weeks. 4 drops a day for 14 days 2 drops for a further 14 days.56+28 = 84. The larger 10 ml bottle 4 drops a day for 14 days and stop. 56. Agreed? Now you really don't have to be a mathematician (!!) To solve this. Guess which bottle has run out? The smaller one, which I need for another 2 weeks. Of course! Plenty of the larger bottle. But I don't need THAT one. You've no idea how tricky it was proving to get more drops. I tried GP but Rottweiler not helpful. I was at the hospital waiting and hoping and waiting…. had to be 'checked first' costing God knows what to check my eyes with groovy equipment. But pleeeeaasse all I needed were some more drops. Please. A great weekend had started, judging by a mass exodus of staff at 16:31...a few hardy patients had stayed on. You really couldn't make it up...a nurse in blue scrubs had wandered in trying to make us all laugh. She'd pinged the reception bell a few times and asking if anyone would like cocktails! Friday the 13th alright. I managed to escape the hospital. I managed to get the bloody drops. Just as the sand – in- my – eye feeling was getting beyond excruciating19:00 Awesome GP Dr Saintly rang me Rottweiler had obviously passed on eye issue to him despite having told me 'Emergencies only' earlier today. 'You, ok?' he asked. 'Bet you need more drops. They NEVER give ANYONE enough I could've done that script earlier today had I known. 'Arghhhh, I wailed...and the bladder? 'I'm on it' he said 'I'll sort it' he said. AT LONG EFFING LAST

38. OPHELIA WEEK, SAT, 21 OCT 2017

Highest wind gust recorded during Storm Ophelia. Roches Point recorded a gust of 155.6km/h on October 16th. A week away in Cornwall. I took my parents, dogs and Daughter 1. You really couldn't make it up. I found Dad lying in a heap, called an ambulance for him. He lay in and on a trolley for hours and hours. No beds. Great staff. Poor staff, how the hell they cope in the chaos of ambulances q queued up outside, no beds inside, photocopying notes. PHOTOCOPYING? That's nuts… where's the technology in that? Puppy got poisoned and he ended up in Vet Hospital. He got a bed within half an hour; vet rang me hourly. Some poor person will have parked in the drop off and found a freezer bag of dog bones which I'd dropped in my haste to get dog out. I can imagine alarm bells as the sight of what looked like human parts and (dog) piddle pewk and whoopsie scattered round the parking space! Eventually we got everyone home late last night thanks to heroic D and my son in law…just as well as I've been throwing up ever since. My mother's effing annoying harp sound on her mobile pinged so much I thought one of us would throw it out the window. Ophelia …more anon…

39. Ophelia part 2, Thu, 26 Oct 2017

There we were back home. Daniel had trained down to West Country. Son-in-law drove through the night to rescue Daughter 1. Daniel then droves non-stop to get my parents' home from a Cornwall break which ended up with Dad in Hospital. In bloody BARNSTAPLE. That architect must be proud of his miserable looking hospital in the middle of nowhere. Where, to park, patients must queue on roundabouts a mile back. Blood pressure must be high by the time they make it if they make it. Puppy Fred. We picked him up en route from his overnight in 'dogspital'…he is ok and recovering from his ordeal with ingested palm oil. The journey home was gruelling. Dad must have been uncomfortable. Daniel's patient. My mother's bloody mobile pinged and ponged a stupid harp sound every time she got a message. I, meanwhile, just could not stop throwing up. With a stabbing pain down my left side, it was a long way home. The pain turned into a sort of smashed glass feeling under my ribs and shaking and shuddering, two duvets and an electric blanket made no difference. Of course, poor Daniel was very worried. He rang Jerome. Hurrah for Jerome, he got me a bed in his London hospital and off we drove once more. Got admitted by a blood stained grumpy RMO: "why are you here" – him. "I'm not well" – me "We have no record of you. But someone with your birthdate was in the hospital last year…. was that you"? "No" I replied "really, if it's easier I'll leave" Somehow it got resolved. Awesome staff nurse and nurse on nights took over. Cannula went in. Chat with Jerome. Meds. Fluids. Bloods etc. etc. Suddenly ok. Next day ditsy day staff did not know I was there, and the intravenous drips etc. ran out at 8. Did not get redone till Daughter 2 turned up at 12:30 and protested to all and sundry. Catering didn't know I was there either they went nuts as I hadn't filled in my 'menus'. "Sorry" I recall muttering. No water jugs. No food …not that I wanted anything. Anyhow, in strode Jerome, calmness personified. Telling funny stories about chain smoking patients trailing catheter bags asunder. He sorted everything. He sorted the meds. Sorted the staff. And it was the weekend. Phew. Order restored. He explained the 'numbers' …50 means you have an infection…no kidding? Sherlock. Fantastic day nurse. She was, utterly OCD. That's brilliant when you are chained to a bed. She insisted on drugs being done to the very second, they ran out. She sorted everything like a military commander. Pushing past Jerome to make sure I got the next stuff on time. No consultant would get in the way of her work! Night staff 2 was hilarious. She'd not been told she was a duty-back-up nurse. Went to the gym and emerged to find 100 missed calls. Managed to nip home. Tell the kids and rush into work.it was late-night getting drugs that night. But when you know why it's fine. We chatted and laughed all night. Her kids turned out to be 30 and 32. There I was worrying they'd been left alone at home; she could go to work to drug me! In fact, I was laughing again when Jerome arrived in the morning. Not seeing the night nurse sorting stuff in the bathroom, he asked if I'd finally lost it…laughing to myself alone. Crazy lady. The cackles that emerged from the bathroom helped him realise all was perfectly fine. 50 shades of infection became 15 shades of infection….so we were on the right track Eventually I got home. I was zonked. But fine. Hey ho. Ophelia. PS Dad recovered well. Puppy Fred too.

Messages:

Oh, Jacq what a story

When things go wrong in a minor way, I get cross and impatient, and then think of your troubles and you always laughing about it. What a ghastly time and journey from Cornwall. You have devised a brilliant mechanism of coping by looking for the humour and then making us all laugh… and weep. I cannot emphasize how much I admire that.

40. Ophelia Part 3 – The clinicians, Thu, 26 Oct 2017

Night nurse1 and I chattered away about storm Ophelia and the devastation that was caused in Ireland. Polite to a fault she even asked me…four hourlies. If it was convenient for ME, for her to do the observations. She was brilliant. Worked out how to spread the painkillers…. thought of everything. Called the kitchen people a walking nightmare when she found out they'd forgotten I was there. Day Nurse was perhaps a bit just a bit, OCD. She was routine obsessed. I loved it.

As for Jerome what can I say? We first met way back when Wingrave, that supremo of all surgeons, demanded he change my stents as an emergency. I'll never forget that first phone call just hours before.

'I've not operated on a patient I've not met!'

Just how he finds the time to make phone calls, let alone make out he's got all the time in the world to listen to a wailing pathetic patient, I really don't know. He's been the same ever since. Keeping an eye on his colleagues. Checking every detail. Forgetting nothing! Advising. Checking. Thinking ahead. Telling funny vomit -from -car stories, leaking -urine-bag stories to keep me giggling! (This was the verb for giggling along). In fact, only that afternoon Jerome had rung. He'd bumped into Dipstick. Updated him. Dip apparently suggested Jerome must be my favourite surgeon now.

Err NOW? Jerome has always been favourite and I gather he told Dipstick as much. Poor old Dipstick he has no bloody idea.

41. Fireworks, Mon, 30 Nov

You'd think, wouldn't you that after the Ophelia saga peace would descend for a bit. You'd maybe think after a spell in hospital bugs would be too scared to emerge. You would think the rest of the family would be fit and well and charging around. Well of course you would be wrong. My parents 60th Anniversary last weekend. Somehow or other everyone turned up. Around the table 50% had visited hospital in the 7 preceding days including Dad, me and daughter-in-law (horse riding accident 22 stitches). Those that had not been medicals that week fell afoul of some dreadful bug in the night. They were all ill in my house. Last guest left Monday. I have been spraying Dettol on every nook and cranny ever since. I never did get the precious script from Jerome. Nor the meds I had left in hospital. Despite 50 Phone calls. As infection started to rage once more, I tried to contact Dipstick. Jerome was away. Dipstick around. His secretary said he'd ring between patients. Then she said he would ring after Clinic. Then she said he'd ring after he operated. Then she said he'd suggested I make an appointment to see him next week. (I already had). I emailed. I texted. I rang. Please help. GP does not have discharge letter. GP needs to know what to do. GP scooped me out of Rottweiler zone, no appointment, and he was meant to be sorting his spreadsheets not patients! He went through everything. Checked measured.

Listened. We need to find out more he said. We tried. He tried. I tried. Bloods, msu, observations…low threshold for readmittance, he said. Mhmm let's talk to London he said. But of course, Dipstick had not replied. Then it was the weekend. The end.

42. The English Patients, Sun, 12 Nov 2017

You may remember that in August I went down to Sussex to stay with my 'living-with-cancer' friend. I call her 'Patsy'. Absolutely Fabulous Patsy. We were meeting for a photo shoot for health and hygiene. The photographer flew in from Sweden. The wonderful awesome 'Pippi' as in Longstocking. Pippi had the unenviable task of capturing our stories in celluloid. Just to add to the pressure, Patsy had just heard she had gone from 'living with' to 'dying with' cancer. I had opened the fizz, we swore like troopers and got on with the shoot. Of course, it was all meant to be about the big 'C' as in CONTINENCE, but the big Cancer way is a more massive story. We promised ourselves we would go to the opening of the photographic exhibition. Patsy promised she would stay alive. Guess what? She did. We did. It was awesome. We wedged flights in between hospital bloods for Patsy. Chemo for Patsy. Appointments for me. We organised assistance at the airport. We were yelled at by the Gatwick Assistance team. They said we were late. They said, 'disabled needed to check in 3 hours before the flight' FFS speeding from hospital to Gatwick, only hand luggage, checked in online….do not shout at us. Just get the bloody wheelchair and golf buggy thing out. We managed somehow. We maybe didn't look like we needed assistance. We bloody well did. Our combined medical accoutrements and metal implants set all the security buzzing! We tweeted a complaint. Gatwick answered. Such was the power of twitter, they rolled out the red carpet on our return!

We were whisked from Stockholm airport to car to hotel. Drinks in the bar. Coats collected for us from our rooms. Little stagger to a recommended restaurant ... lager, schnapps, and shrimps. What more could we possibly want? All the groovy people of Stockholm were there. Turns out it was a sort of Soho style; edgy epicentre trendy meets sultry beatnik bastion. We loved it. Bet Stieg Larsson went there. We were met next morning by our lovely host Mr B. We have decided to adopt him. He was Danish. He was utterly wonderfully open, direct, funny and bucketful of emotional intelligence. He whisked us by taxi and lift, to the tallest building in Stockholm. He had a fixed table for lunch. There you see, he said. All of Stockholm from the comfort of your seat. What a hero. We would never have made it otherwise. Our creaking bodies...trying to keep up. Then off we whizzed to the opening of the exhibition. Patsy's photo was up there in big focus. She did her interview, she smiled radiantly, and she looked amazing. Pippi arrived. We hugged. We cried. Her parents, husband, tiny daughter. They hugged us too. *So, you are the famous English patients*. Her mother said.... We grinned. We laughed. We showed off our best Swedish: '.*Tak*'. '*Hey*'. When we were not sure we went for '.*Hurdy Gurdy*'. Then after the compulsory fizz...we let rip with our knowledge of '.The Bridge.' Then just to show off...'. Where was the girl with the Dragon Tattoo?' Just when we were really becoming crazier than normal...we announced we must leave for the airport.

Oh no...they implored...the speeches? The panel discussion? The canapés? We need you. Ever direct...Patsy pronounced. *Sorry got to go.... Chemo in the morning...got to dash.* .... Off we went.... Barely 24 hours after our arrival. Back to Gatwick and the red carpet. Asleep by midnight. Back to our various hospitals next morning. Aching screaming bodies. But bugger that.... We had had a 'blast'. We will be back...Patsy has promised to stay alive...we looked forward to the New York opening. See you there...*Hey Hey*!! **Messages**:

HOPE AND POWER. *Dear English Ladies.......It was such an honour to have you coming to the exhibition. It meant a lot to me; I would have loved to spend more time together. Thank you much for your lovely words and for you letting me picture you. Kind of you to bring a gift for my daughter, she said the night after "I want to read Winniw (sic) the Pooh" and her daddy translated! My parents really enjoyed meeting you, and they told me they think your both are lovely. They are not that good in English but really appreciate your chat! I am happy I had the chance to get to know you both! You. Give hope and power. Warm regards and love,'Pippi'.*

WHAT A BLAST: Dear *Ladies! What a blast I had with you, and I was super happy that you came. Hope the flight went well and they treated you like princesses this time! ...Our CEO mentioned your images in the panel debate and the chat you had with him. I will send you the video compilation and later on the digital exhibition but that will be in December. And then we stay in touch for sure, these meetings are worth a lot. And all the best tomorrow and onwards with the chemo's* *and treatment. I count on good progress reports! Big hug from me and super nice to meet and spend time. We'll stay in touch! Mr B*

Email

Wow, this was truly impressive and inspiring. Well done. What a journey, what an adventure and what a story. But you did it. Hope you are recovering… you brave ladies. Very proud to know you…Bee.

43. Piddle and Patsy, Sun, 19 Nov 2017

Since then Patsy had been pewking and I had been neuking. To explain. Patsy + Chemo = pewk. We had swapped tons of jolly banter to distract. Patsy was a bit better and wrote a piece for a magazine to accompany the 'Stockholm Pippi Photos'. Meanwhile, I had many communications with Dip. Having sworn I would never ever see him EVER again on account of the disasters of the last weeks. He rang. Shock. He apologised. Shock. He explained his office was in disarray. He explained he had expected to see me. In fact, he had me listed for 3 appointments in one clinic. (No surprises there, it **was** customary to tell the patient she has an appointment!) He suggested I see him the very next day. I relented. I went. He was not late, well only 20 minutes. He did remember my name. He organized nuclear imaging. Whoooo Hoooo. Hence the neuking. A bit of CT imaging too just for good measure. A bit of resetting of the SNS implant too. His last effort seemed to make my toes curl, shock! He has appealed to the rep again. I then saw him again the next week. He didn't quite get my name right, but nearly, never mind. He was tired. He yawned a lot. No stifle, just big old, tired yawns. Am I really that boring? He also, banged his head on his desk in frustration that I appear to have another infection. That was ok, I think. At least he understands. I feel like banging my head on a weekly basis…. Would this be his version of empathy?

I also met a colleague of his. An amazing awesome lovely lady doctor. Honestly, you'd think we'd known each other for years. We quickly covered old ground, we giggled about Dipstick (she'd been at a dinner with him) but of course she said, *what happens on a dinner stays on a dinner*! The mind boggles. She was groovy. She was innovative. She had an idea, how about iv at home wow…keep me out of hospital plan…….but we will have to wait for NHS-land to organise it…could be next year some time. No rush then. She even asked me how I managed to get from home to the clinic, when I am feeling so crap. She seems to care…like in bucketfuls. It really helped. It was the little things. She also remembered my name. #Not rocket science Oh and as I left for Dip's clinic…she called out….'. *Give 'Dipstick' a kiss*!' I grinned and yelled back *'YOU MUST BE BLOODY JOKING'*…. goodness knows what the assembled bladder patients waiting outside thought…. Did I care? Not a jot…So I was once more waiting for results…antibiotics…and innovation…

Email from a friend

Oh dear Jacq, this does not sound very good. You'll need to stop pewking before Xmas and all that booze. It must be hell feeling ill. You are making friends right left and centre and at least some of them are looking after you and trying to make things better. Fingers crossed. You must feel like screaming and weeping all too often, and still manage to make us laugh. I salute you. A big hug.

44. Jam pots, Sat, 25 Nov 2017

In the race to get the latest test results NHS London Hospital won. I had 'unknown' phone call Monday.

Nurse: *You have infection.*

Me: *No surprise there* ("Sherlock")

Me: *What's the antibiotic sensitivities, please?*

Nurse: *Resistance to Nitro and CoAmox*

Me: *Ah those are the ones I've been on. What can I use instead?*

Nurse: *I'll ask Consultant*

Me: *Great. When?*

Nurse: *when I see her…….next week*

ME: *oh. How about your email the results to me?*

Nurse: *mm I cannot do that without admin support. …. pause…. silence…. I can fax your GP.*

Me: ***@@'*

Dipstick's Office came a close second. When I rang (as instructed). They said they were understaffed very busy and would try to find the results. Me: **@@' In the end only 8 days after I needed it Jerome had once again sailed into battle. Got a script sent to my chemist. Albeit FFFF FAX …took THREE DAYS!? And have gone back onto pewkville antibiotics. Frrrrr.

Dipstick? Not a word. He is probably yawning.

Meanwhile I somehow got to a House of Commons APPG (Continence) Committee Awesome. I was sensible …well, a couple of slip ups… I asked the Prof.

Chairperson of Royal College of GPs why msu pots were rationed by receptionists trained in the Rottweiler school of gate keeping. After all I asked. What do you think we are going to do with the pots? Make bloody jam? I further suggested patients generally could help here. How about we buy our own. As I have now found Amazon £5 for 50.

You cannot do that. She spoke. Shock horror. *They might not be the right shape to catch pee and fit the lab machine.*

Me: **@@

What else. The updated and edited by me...NHS Guidance about to come out. We have worked hard on that. Our chairperson was there to explain. She was fab. All credit to her for getting it sorted. A GP spoke about his surgery in London having an evidence gathering RCT based on NHS 2015 Guide recommendations, Focus on frail elderly. I asked if not frail not elderly could be included. I did allude to our eBay system of booking GP appointments. Ooops. Should not have done that. My neighbour nudged me….and whispered I cannot believe you said that. Ooooopppss. Alas we missed our train but … perchance the station forecourt was launching a fizzy snowy drink show. It would have been rude to rush past. Wrapped in bright orange blankets, we sipped fizz out of bright orange glasses, watched the snow and grinned. Nearly missed the next train too!

45. Hallelujah, Sat, 16 Dec 2017

The last couple of weeks had been a bit of a blur. Bladder buggerations. Dipstick gone AWOL. His office has gone tits up. Then awesome Jerome trying valiantly to cover-up and help. Another infection with some Sci-Fi sounding bug has hit. Jerome tentatively suggested IV. I could not reply. Bladder implant I have switched off. Dipstick needs to work out if the leads have migrated. The rep asked him, I asked him. No response.

Normally I write this Daily Stent to absorb my screams of frustration. My incandescent swearing. But hark, a tad earlier than expected a tiny little person has arrived. Daughter 1 who has had unbelievably traumatic time for the last 7 years, has safely and brilliantly got herself through this next stage of her young life. Her story was not mine to tell. I can tell you though, that I cannot shout, or swear, or frankly move. I have been to Mothercare so many times the assistant knows be by name. Sainsbury's helped me to my car because my shopping revealed my new status, (the discount bottle of champagne, nestled in the nappies, gave it away). This new status must be etched on my face, as I have been offered a seat on a train AND a tube. Unheard of. Whilst trying to stuff antibiotics all I need to do was hold on to this wonderful little baby, type with one finger and try to forget the rubbishness of bugs in bladders, kicking kidney, screaming spine and dopey Dipstick.

Email from a friend:

Most of this was wonderful. I cannot believe you are making light of all your troubles and thank God for this precious new life to cheer up the bad times. Crossing my fingers for a happy pain free, drama less Christmas for you all, you deserve it.

And to all a good night Thu, 28 Dec 2017

'Twas the week before Christmas.

Not a creature was sleeping, at all. In our house.

The nappies all stacked by the bin with due care.

The baby was hungry, his mum was too.

Son 2 had one of his heads…

I had my meds ……. I will stop there, terrible lines It's been fun. We have provided bed and full board, washing, cooking, wines, carol singing. …. In scenes I'm sure repeated in all your homes too. Happy Christmas to all and to all a good night!

46. A LANDMARK STEP IN LOCAL GP SERVICES! WED, 03 JAN 2018

It had been a good week. Upper and lower uti been burbling away. I persuaded Rottweiler to send an msu off. The practice was now part of a new merged group. Promising and I quote:' a landmark step in the development of services in our area… '…I rang this super-duper new service. After no less than 2 hours continuous trying I managed to get through to the reception Rottweiler. Rottweiler could only tell me the result was back and was:

'As expected,' and added, 'I am not trained to give out results.

A landmark step? Pleeeassseee just tell me what it says…I gave up when she stuttered over the medical terms…'red blood cells…. white cells…elliptical cells……?? @@@@~~~~

In addition. My phone had had an infection…it delayed messages. So, just when I thought I had got memory loss and wrote another, it sent ten at once. I sent apologies to anyone who had been hit by my messages. But help was at hand. Phone chat online thingy told me how to sort. Think I have done it. Then, I had an asthma check. To get repeat prescriptions for asthma it was necessary to book a spurious appointment with the nurse. I can book an appointment. Then get a script for puffer online. Then cancel the appointment and that way get my script. Bonkers. But I had forgotten to cancel this one which I'd booked 3 months ago. I went. Saw the nurse I have known for years. (Taught her children at school). We chatted about her family's Christmas. My family. My bladder! Explained about swimming in lakes being better than public pools. She laughed loudly when I explained why! Leaky bladder! Sped through the statutory asthma questionnaire.

'Can you breathe'? Answer: yes.

Asked her to print my msu result. Of course, she said. We looked at it together. Why on earth the Rottweiler could not have at least read it on the phone I do not know. It did have the 'sensitivities 'on it, after all. Much for her denials. Some resistant pewky bug this one. I will have to go to plan B. On Monday. So, using up the nurse's valuable appointment slot. I have given her a giggle. Got my msu result. Oh, and can have puffers if needed for the next year. Bloody bonkers system.

Meanwhile I have tweeted and written to the President of GPs in England. I met her at the House of Commons last year. I asked her then to use reception staff to support GPs. They could really be trained along with all support staff to, well SUPPORT. Or at least give out standard test results, sample pots and well just be **nice**! I had not heard from Uncle Montmorency about promised rescheduled appointments. 'I will ring you first thing tomorrow 'his secretary had said on Wednesday, as I nearly boarded my train. Dipstick has moved to a new office. Not answering phones or emails... I would not blame them for having me on their 'ignore' list. Jerome had again offered to help. He was hoping to get paperwork sorted so that I could send msu to the lab without hassling anyone.

47. Bingo, Thu, 11 Jan 2018

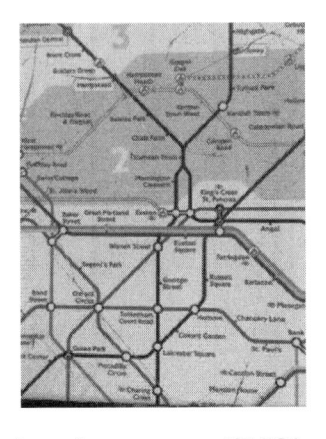

I keep seeing the same man on trains he is very nice. I think he is a friend of Daniel but I'm too embarrassed to ask him his name. Daniel thinks he works at GCHQ. Maybe he wants me to do a secret mission. He would be surprised if he tried to follow me…. Way back in 2017!! You may recall I was having trouble with the bladder implant known as 'SNS'. After a series of frustrations Dipstick …tried to reprogram it and then the SNS Rep cancelled her appointment to try to fix it. Dipstick was going to 'write a strongly worded letter to the company' (bet he did not). Anyhow I switched SNS off as it appeared to be stimulating my toes rather than bladder. Toes great. Bladder not great. After a bit of head scratching managed to get an appointment with the SNS nurse. His name I could not fathom. But it sounds like Bingo. And there I was 3 months later headed for London once more en route I'd arranged to collect precious 'forms' from Jerome's new quarters. (JHQ). Arrived at JHQ….no forms…everyone looked blankly at me as though I had lapsed into Russian code. Never mind I burbled….and I wandered off to the next hospital to see Bingo. By utter awesome bloody brilliance, my old friend and original SNS nurse was doing a one-off Clinic. Let us call her, 'legs eleven'. Maternity 'keeping in touch'. Wow I said unbelievable luck for me. She was thorough. She was honest. She knows all the men in my boat. She understands! Turns out the SNS was not working. (Really Sherlock?) The SNS had been reCAS-programmed. And the leads seem to have migrated. To stimulate the spinal nerve. I.e., toe curling. Leg banging agony. What to do? Better see one of the men in the boat. But which one? As for the forms.... well if I had a GPS tracker it would look something like this....my Fitbit (fitbitch as D calls it) went into overdrive and as I type on my train, it informs me I am an overachiever! Jerome ended up meeting me, in the street. As you do, finding the forms himself, in JHQ and leaping back to consultant tasks at his hospital.... If the Russians had been tracking us, they would surely have got confused! Thank goodness for Jerome. As for Bingo I've still no idea who on earth he was. Who cares? Legs Eleven Made in Heaven....

48. Uncle to the Rescue, Wed, 17 Jan 2018

Bad bugs on the rampage. I got a text message from the new' super-duper GP surgery. 'Ring surgery for your latest test results 'I did. Rottweiler receptionist responded eventually. Of course, she would not give me result. As in: she withheld my result. Told me I had to make a phone appointment with a doctor. Unspecified time. Tomorrow. Previous experience in this ridiculousness has given me the strategies …. I drove to the surgery and requested a printout of my latest results. This usually works well. Not today. The new lady on reception said she would print it. She printed pages and pages which turned out to be a list of all tests since 2oo8…lots of paper but NO RESULTS. Ffs. GP Saint P (no pun intended) had seen me in his reception. What a hero. He rang me and asked if I was ok. I explained. He was bloody nice told me to go back and he would see me. But of course, I had a train to catch. I said I was fine and thank you. I arrived to see Uncle Montmorency microbiology, but I had NO results to show him. Uncle greeted me with a massive bear hug and a cough. Up the stairs we clomped. He in his biker boots… he had had a bad flu bug. (The last appointment had been cancelled as I boarded the train). He admitted to opting for the wrong flu vaccine for himself. Now, he should know better! Uncle listened, explained, made me laugh, he has a better lab with a better form to get a better result. Perhaps ANY result. He did a brilliant impression of Dipstick banging his head on his desk muttering.

49 Chocolate, Sat, 20 Jan 2018

No further news. No results. No nothing. Radio silence from the doctors in the boat. I was pouring in anything I could think of and hoping Uncle Montmorency will be in touch.... pleeeeaaasssseee. Could not stop sneezing. Uncles' flu bugs or, (more likely) allergy to hyacinths I encountered yesterday. Seriously, for some reason they make me sneeze. Quite apart from all this, there had been an interesting exchange on twitter. Aimed at surgeons. They were discussing allergies. Contrast dye allergy. I discovered I was allergic to that when this all began. I declare it at check in for every procedure. The lack of transferable notes between hospitals, doctors and patients means the patient must coordinate the information. Of course, the doctor must trust/ believe the patient. If she says she is allergic she probably was allergic. The twitter feed was interesting because this was not generally understood. This reminded me of one of my spinal procedures. I told admitting nurse, other nurses, anaesthetwast, and theatre staff, everyone, that I was allergic to contrast dye. The put a red band on my wrist. ALLERGIC. The surgeon had operated on me many times. Never one to make eye contact or small talk he clearly knew' best.... he used ....CONTRAST...... I had reacted badly, as in anaphylactic badly, ooops... maybe patients sometimes do know something? Why am I allergic? Goodness only knows.

50. Nice waiting rooms, Sun, 28 Jan 2018

How many hours does a patient spend waiting in waiting rooms? My GP surgery specialises in training the receptionists. They follow the Rottweiler training method. This makes for a confrontational approach. The line across the floor, indicating the border controls. Do not step over this until invited to approach the reception desk. The fact that 1 metre in front of the ever-seething queue, the previous patient interrogation can be heard verbatim. Privacy, eh? Imagine my surprise then when I had occasioned this week to visit my daughter's surgery. There was NO stupid border line marked out. The receptionists follow the Labrador School method. Be nice, be intelligent, bit of a chatter and ooze empathy. 'N.I.C.E.' They explained the GP was running late. They said there had been two emergencies which had caused the delays. They suggested patients could come back a bit later or see the nurse or the pharmacist or book ahead. They offered water to drink, changing rooms for babies to be fed. They held babies for parents. In fact, they appeared to rather WANT to be nice. Everyone was calm, happy, and chatty. What a difference. I also had a check-up in the London hospital eye clinic. This was always slow, but the patients are given eye drops to dilate and. This means no one can see. Yellow tears drip down faces and everyone (I am the youngest by about 25 years) nods off snoring away. Yes, I did that too. There was no need for the TV with subtitles on the wall. We CANNOT see! Two and a half hours later Consultant saw me. Apologised profusely for delays. Explained reasons. Spent ages. Thorough. Showed me scans. Explained the technology. Intelligence. Chatter. Empathy. Nice. I staggered out peering at my phone to ring for a cab.

Then there are the waiting rooms at St Pancras. One was conveniently by Eurostar and East Midlands Trains. After all these bloody appointments I get an East Midlands train…one day I might just get the Paris one!! This waiting room has staff trained the NICE way. There was a button to press for champagne. There was a button to press for a heater. Phone charger point. It is an excellent waiting room. Especially with the benefits of a founding member loyalty card! NICE…I will meet you there…anytime!

51. Waiting Room part 2, Tue, 30 Jan 2018

A train to London. Met my truly awesome friend DG …we found seats…in first class…. chattered all the way and no one asked us to pay. Scurried past Waiting Room. Got to appointment. Consultant 'Wingrave the one who tells everyone he was actually the BEST. Had not arrived. He eventually did. Saw another patient before me. BUGGER. Saw Wingrave he was on broadcast mode. I could not get a word in edgeways. I sprinted back to the station. I missed my train by 3 minutes. Went down the escalator to get some water… with a thud a crash and a yell the passenger behind let go of her massive suitcase. It tumbled down, hit me and we all ended in a heap at the bottom. No worries. I am fine. Bruises that is all. Got next train. I was only 20 minutes late for my Tuesday teaching. BAN ALL WHEELIE SUITCASES…

52. Naked surgeon, Sat, 03 Feb 2018

As for the trauma of the tourist throwing her large pink suitcase down the escalator at me. (I was seriously ok. Awesome lovely ski-chatter-physio has checked me out...neck was the only pain. As in Pain in the Neck). Taking distraction in reading I have been lent a book called the Naked Surgeon. Sounds dodgy! But it was in fact written by a friend of and a dedication to, my cardiologist neighbour. The subject matter was in fact health economics. I have been getting my head round the data gathering, evidence-based practice to make sense of NICE guidelines. In my naivety I thought adverse events were death ...but no... It could be excessive bleeding. Aha. That was personally significant and takes me back to 2009. The book was very readable...honestly!! I particularly liked a reference to 'eminence based surgeons'....a type of surgeon who likes to take risks and believes that evidence based medicine was like painting by numbers for pedestrian artists, but not for him, self-styled da Vinci that he or she was ...and eminence-based medicine was defined as persisting in making the same mistakes over and over again, with ever increasing conviction. This was insane. I was so irritable. Discombobulated...needed to find...more humour I would find that when I found my mojo.

53. Fri, 09 Feb 2018 Willy Wonka

Another great week in bladder lands. Some 3(!) years ago Jerome suggested I get myself onto the waiting list of a surgeon in London who 'does infections.' Well somehow or other I did just that. Saw her first in 2016. Tricky to get appointments but.... Second appointment was 2017. She's great, nice intelligent chatter empathy NICE. By amazing luck, I was contacted by her hospital telling me I had another appointment this week. That is like getting the golden ticket to Wonka's chocolate factory. A Roald Dahl prize winning ticket to Hospital. Back on the bloody train again.... The reason? The appointment was to a joint consultation with both consultant and her colleague consultant microbiologist. Two doctors one patient. They were brilliant. YUSS new ideas, new plan. It was agony going over the story again. Why do you only have one kidney? Why did you have a bladder reconstruction ...once? Twice? THREE times? Why did you have stents? Why are you allergic? What are you allergic to? And the interrogation went on.... arrrrghhhhhh. Whilst waiting for the appointment. I stood by the bin, as usual. The waiting room never has enough chairs. In any case I hate the effing loud TV blaring out Brexit news...and my spine was better upright. A kind man offered me his seat and thanking him profusely I declined. Whilst waiting, young be-suited doctor came out of his room. He knocked on another room and a very important looking purple scrubs-clad doctor came out. They spoke urgently about his patient. A worry about the poor man's private parts. The discussion was of course overheard by the WHOLE waiting room. Having planned, they busily returned to their rooms. Of course, we all tried not to look up as the hapless patient emerged from his appointment. Poor man. WillieWonkie. Ouch. Was this breach of confidentiality? Yes of course it was. The assumption from the doctors that we patients were sitting there deaf and blind and brain dead. We could hear every word. Just like when the cubicle curtains are drawn on a ward. For privacy? The good thing was patients are pretty good at not saying anything. What happens in Hospital stays in Hospital.

In the book I have just been loaned by cardiologist neighbour 'Naked Surgeon'. The fact that there are many people in the operating theatre was a moot point. If all goes well i.e., the patient lives. And the 'team' did well. If not, and for cardio that is a binary situation ...i.e., dies...the surgeon takes the blame. That is brutal. No amount of consent forms can ever make up for it. Despite all my whinging I have the greatest respect for surgeons. What responsibility what courage.

*In a strange parallel I should explain that Son 2 known as BFG, was born with a heart defect. In many hours, nights, days, years, of hospitalisation looking out over the Thames, there are many memories I would rather forget. My decision to consent to a drug was one story. The surgeon carefully explained possible side effects to me. He then moved to the next sick baby and of course I could hear every word of the same conversation. Even though the privacy curtains were drawn. Nervously I chose to accept the treatment plan for BFG. He improved and we got home in time for Christmas. The baby next to us did not have the drug. He got sicker. He did not go home for Christmas. The long list of possible side effects included: stunted growth. As Son2 was now fit and well and at 6'6" a keen sportsman. I am glad I signed the consent form.

54. Minority Report or bionic robotics, Tue, 20 Feb 2018

Minority Report. *Hello. As I write I am lying on a hospital bed. Do not panic. All ok. My spinal implant was not working.*

I had rung the special Hospital number for bionic patients. That was last week messaging machine told me I should get a response within 7 days or ring again 'in case the message had been mislaid'!? I tried the special email too. That auto reply said I should get a response from the 'team' within 5 working days. Sensing this endless loop was loopy I braved up and … I tried the lovely rep's secret number. She replied immediately. She is left the company, but the London rep would be in touch. He was. He organized. He had me in here within 12 hours. I cancelled today's maths and awesome Patsy who was visiting was holding the home front. I am hoping she will be updating me on Elise Christie at the Winter Olympics. Or maybe best not know. I was even expected by the jolly receptionist. I was quickly ushered into a room in a dark basement along the Euston Road. And my bionics were being sorted as I typed. The room lights were on an NHS eco setting they had automatically turned off and I did not have the encoder to turn them back on. Hence iPad was in use! There was even a very groovy ceiling light auto thing to stare at through the darkness. It could be a sky above a beach somewhere. Cannot find Tom Cruise yet but he's probably on a pre crime program chip trip.

55. Bilbo Baggins, Thu, 22 Feb 2018

I had been reprogrammed. I had new charger kit. I was plugged in and slowly spine was improving. I was supposed to have telephone follow up call with the Bingo nurse. This was to update on the bladder implant progress or lack of. As in the leads had migrated which meant nerve pathways shockingly painful if implant was on... Keep by your phone half an hour before and half an hour after the appointment time, warned my letter and text. I did. 29 minutes AFTER my time slot my phone rang. Hello this was Bingo from London. I have a call booked with you. I am afraid I'm too busy to speak to you.! £££that is that then! In other news I had another appointment booked with Uncle Montmorency...at his behest.... but his secretary has emailed. He was not doing that clinic anymore. Great. That is that cancelled too. Then because I have another msu result urgently needed, and really, I have nothing better to do than make medical calls or wait in all day, I rang for that. The answer message said press 1 for Bilbo 2 for Baggins and 3 Frodo. I chose 1. Got some inane music and then of course went straight to some crap message 'all our lines are busy please leave a message after the tone. 'So, I did. No response'.

Olympics had been good, hadn't it? Suddenly, we were curling experts again, 4 years after our last episode! Sweeping the kitchen floor was cool again. Clare Balding doing great in Salford (took me a while to realise she was not actually in Korea!)

56. FARTED AND LEFT THE ROOM, THU, 01 MAR 2018

I had managed to get the spinal implant running again. Last week's sorties into hospitals continued. But by the next Friday, my spine was a lot better, but kidney was grumbling. In truth it had been all week but got muddled with the spine bits. In trying to get the latest msu by phone and email but not managed anything but out-of-office replies. I had not wanted to disturb Jerome all week, but I ended up buggering up his weekend. He found results. Speedily. Why the hell can no one else do that? He then explained that 'R' next to every antibiotic on the results meant Resistance and perhaps an IV in hospital would be best course of action. Leaving a snoring Daniel on the sofa, I started to assemble a bag of overnight bits…i.e., implants, chargers, drugs and iPad! Slept badly and broke the news to poor Daniel at 6 next morning. Hospital nurses greeted me like a long-lost friend. They have the 'N.I.C.E.' protocol in bucket loads. Nice. Intelligence. Care. Empathy. Made decisions fast. Jerome kept me up to speed by text (how inclusive did that feel) and visits. Sunday, he instructed a trip outside…rather than a jumping out of the window as I had suggested. Littlest son (BFG) and I tripped out and pretended to buy out some groovy techie shop. All those groovy gadgets one could not exist without. We tried to get a coffee in a healthy kitchen place. I say tried because

BFG only wanted tap water and spinach pie, I only wanted tap water and coffee. Water with a sprig of mint in it was £5.95. The staff insisted we had to have salad and resisted our attempts to say no. We ended up with much bloody natural rabbit food we popped it in a takeaway box. Chickpeas a plenty. Farty reported BFG. We gave the takeaway to Daniel when he arrived later. 'Got your supper for you' we said! Daughter 2 popped in and out in between work and rowing and coughing and buying Nature's Kitchen skinny flat white coffee for me! Drips, and TV, and nurses especially at night making me laugh and telling me anecdotes of the olden days. Did you know? They said, we used to do knitting at night! Now we must be busy looking after patients (novel) and when we are not busy, we must do online CPD. If we don't, we get rude messages telling us we will not get paid.... Wow I said ...I better tell the teachers I know. I was freezing cold one minute boiling the next. I had to answer stupid bloody questions...what allergies? Loads...when did this start? 2009...I just handed sheets of my notes hastily printed at home. Or maybe that was an old teaching plan? Oh well same difference. Objectives. Impacts. Immeasurability. Reflective journal (what-a-load of bollocks). Monday I was wheeled off for a scan. They kept insisting I should have a full bladder but seeing as I waited from 9.00 am to 15.00 I kind of got passed off (literally..., bladder has no stop function you see!!). The radiology lady eventually turned up. Dragged me backwards on the wheelchair of joy. She wheeled me into the scanner room. Left me there in darkness. I found myself staring at a be-anoraked little lady staring at a screen. She muttered away, ran out, (what did I say?) came back with the radiology lady and then started the scan. She farted questions at me. (This was a word I have made up...it was from the verb to start to fire) | *You need a CT? Do I?* Err?? Presumably Jerome was the judge of that? *Where was your right kidney? Why did you lose it?* (Silly me) Why could I not empty my bladder? Why did I have a bladder reconstruction...? argghghghgh? *Excuse me, I said.... but who are you?* She muttered. *Dr Baggage face* and then told me to hold my breath. I did...for ages and ages and ages until I simply could not hold it anymore. ...Pahe buggered up her images. she farted more questions, muttered about a CT and scuttled out of the room...

Whilst in hospital I rang to cancel things, not least my renal appointment. Annual check-up on the 6th anniversary of losing, carelessly, the right kidney. The call handler told me that I would lose my place in the waiting list if I cancelled again. I am sorry, I said, I will try not to be in hospital, again. I got no response to that. Uncle Montmorency rang today. His secretary had scheduled that for 17.15. He rang at 17.50. But he rang to say he was ringing in between patients, and he had another patient now and rang off. I get that I am low on his list too!! Then once I was home, I rang GP as instructed by hospital, to ask for potassium stuff which apparently, I need. They rang back later insisting they needed instructions in writing from Jerome. I told them not to worry I would eat bananas and tomatoes from Tesco instead. The

Rottweiler laughed at that!!! Cow! Now what? Dunno. I will see Jerome, if I ever get through to a human voice to make an appointment and he will I am sure come up with a plan or at least make me laugh.

57. Tough. Shit. Thu, 29 Mar 2018

March was meant to be sunny. It snowed.

We were meant to have a week's holiday. We cancelled.

I was supposed to be teaching on Tuesdays. I managed none….

It all started well. A 24-hour trip to Dublin. This was an education programme day for clinicians the male/female psyche for motivational interviewing. In short, persuading patients to use CISC. That is: clean intermittent self-catheterisation. My fellow patient was an awesome young man who broke his back skiing in the Antarctic. He has taught me much. He refuses to 'battle' he refuses to be 'bound' …. Wheelchair bound he was NOT. He was wheelchair **enabled** strong. His progress through airport security proved his point, he sped through. Laughing at my interrogation and personal searches by the guards! Disposable catheters, bionic metal body and bags of antibiotics always cause a scene for me! I returned home coughing and sneezing blaming the snow and lack of Guinness. Cutting a very long story short for two weeks I was in and out of GP surgery. On the phone to GPs and trying to persuade Rottweiler on the phone, to assist. My breathless phone calls won me a much-prized appointment… to see a duty nurse… she was worried, plugged me into a nebuliser and said she'd get a doctor to assist. Unfortunately, no doctor appeared.

She gave up on that idea and sent me to get a chest X-ray at the hospital. She instructed me to buy a nebuliser and take steroids. She told me my X-ray results would be available in five weeks. Thinking five weeks was a bit (?) long to wait I contacted Surgeon Saint Jerome for help. Jerome-to-the-rescue AGAIN! 24 hours later I was seen by his recommended respiratory consultant friend and promptly admitted to hospital in London. In my wheezy state I walked there. But no one said otherwise.

I just kept walking. Jerome was aghast! Text exchange read something like this:

- Me: I'm walking round now
- Jerome: They made you walk?
- Me: I'm tough
- Jerome: Shit
- Me: Hah
- Jerome: Yeah
- Jerome: Wow...!

My bed for the night was in ITU. My own personal nurses, doctors, inches away leaping to soothe my every cough wheeze and sneeze. And tea too. Nice.

Meanwhile, sadly, my mother-in-law had died totally unexpectedly, in her sleep. Not only ringing my own GP, as above, I was also ringing Scottish GP to agree the death certificate details, undertakers and florists too. Trying to comfort my children and husband with wheezy lungs and spinning head. I wrote the funeral service in hospital. We went over the eulogy after watching the rugby ...in hospital. A few days later I was sufficiently oxygenated to get my release papers. With masses of support and advice from Jerome, off we set for Scotland. We gave One Fine Lady one helluva send off. This added layer of complexity makes us the stronger. We're Tough. Shit. Hah. Yeah. Wow.

58. THE FIRST DECADE

That was my story up until March 2018. Bladderless, kidney less and spineless...as such. The story from 2009 had moved at pace. Leaving teaching, joining NHS patient advocacy conference speaker House of Commons, Lords and Westminster Hall were the venues. I had been awarded the LUTS[33] patient champion award, I wrote my blog, and tweets and appeared on radio and tv. My frustration was and is, I was still struggling health was but also still struggling to raise awareness, change attitudes and improve care for all patients of whatever age. As I have often said, if we could get patients assessed, treated and looked after we would in fact save money. It was not about how many pads to give leaking bladders or bowels. It was about how we might ditch the pads altogether. The adverts extolling the virtues of high absorbency incontinence pads. OOPS moments or not...it was not normal. We need to make sure everyone knows that. It may well be treatable. Ask your GP for a referral to the continence service, or as those are few and far between, a women's health physio, a urologist...get

---

[33] LUTS Lower Urinary Tract

help. Wave the Excellence in Continence Care Guidance[34] at them. Wave the NICE[35] guideline at them.

As I write the last bit of my story so far, I add some answers to many questions from friends and colleagues.

Why?

I did write to the original surgeons the Urological Surgeon and Gynaecologist. I simply asked for their explanations. I received no reply. I then contacted a legal team who offered to help me find out what had happened. They suggested a no-win-no-fee arrangement. I was only looking for answers. Lawyers' letters went back and forth and eventually the operation notes were released. The Urological one simply stated the ureter was obstructed. The Boari flap was formed.

The Gynaecological one was illegible it was unreadable. There then followed another court order requesting transcription. That eventually arrived. The notes were standard but did mention excessive bleeding around the bladder.

The lawyers sought experts to review the notes. None felt able to say anything more than the treatment was substandard. I wondered did they not feel able to do anything more than protect their colleagues, close ranks? Running out of statutory time the lawyers and I agreed to stop, draw a line under it all and move on. The Consult-

---

[34] Excellence In Continence Care Guidance 2015 refreshed 2018 (EICC) https://www.england.nhs.uk/publication/excellence-in-continence-care/.
[35] National Institute for health Care and Excellence (Nice) https://www.nice.org.uk/guidance/ng123.

ants indeed moved on. One retired. The other moved to another area. In truth it probably no longer matters. What on earth happened? Why the delays? Missed diagnoses?

The Consequences

The consequences of all that happened are listed brutally on every letter from the surgeons. The most recent letter has no less than 30 Diagnoses in the opening paragraph. These include boari flap reimplantation, boari flap reconstruction, nephrectomy, L4 L5 spinal fusion, sacral nerve stimulator implantation, recurrent urinary tract infections, 4 hourly self-catheterisations, implantation of L3 to L5 Nevro spinal cord stimulator, suprapubic catheter insertions, suprapubic catheter removals, cystoscopy, L4 L5 S1 spinal injections…I could go on but this was essentially as good as summary as it gets.

Consent

As for consent forms. I simply do not know how a patient can possibly make informed consent minutes before going down to the operating theatre.

I have no recollection of the consent for hysterectomy, I am sure I was told and signed minutes before the operation.

For the first Boari Flap operation I recall asking if the surgeon had ever done such an operation before. The reply was that it was very rare for any surgeon. To do such an operation. Did that mean no? I was also told that he did not know what he would find when he opened me up so it was not clear what the operation would be.

At no time did I realise there was no ICU in the local private hospital, nor did I realise that this could have serious consequences.

I have no recollection of any Multi-Disciplinary Team involvement.

As consultants are not usually employed by the private hospitals and have their own arrangements for clinical indemnity (UK GOV 2020).[36] This seems to indicate that The medical defence unions then seem to be unregulated. Patients would not know this, nor would patients realise the implication.

Before the spinal operations I was verbally told the many problems that might occur during and after surgery. I was given physical hard copies of information packs. I was told to avoid 'googling' but to ask. A second appointment was then made for this and for the signing of consent. On the operation day this consent was again produced read and checked. This of course took up a lot of time for both patient and consultant. For urological procedures, in London I have had the good fortune to be able to ask by email, phone and face to face about consent. Indeed, I a multi surgeon meeting prior to a big operation in 2015, scared both Daniel and me. As did the nephrectomy preadmission warnings. But there have been many occasions where this has simply not hap-

---

[36] UK GOV 2020 Paterson Inquiry https://www.gov.uk/government/publications/paterson-inquiry-report accessed 6 February 2020.

pened. I do not know the answer. I just put it out there. What can be done?

In February 2020 the Paterson Inquiry was released. This related to a surgeon performing in the private sector. Whilst the detail is not relevant to me, personally, the recommendations are:

- The need for a repository of surgeons, private and NHS.
- The need for MDT in both settings
- For writing to the patient and copy to GP rather than the other way round
- The need for transparency and communication between NHS and Private
- The need for regulation of Clinical Indemnity in the independent sector.
- The need to let patients know how complaints may be made via the Parliamentary and Health Service Ombudsman for NHS patients, and via the Independent Sector Complaints Adjudication Service for private.

No wonder my complaints fell on deaf ears. I got absolutely nowhere by writing to the NHS hospital, the private hospital nor the surgeons.

Private Health Insurance

A word about NHS vs Private. Right at the start of this, NHS Urological surgeon moved me from NHS to private across town. It was fortunate indeed that through

Daniel's work, we pay a considerable annual sum for me to have private health insurance cover. Private health care was quicker and held in more luxurious surroundings. But as Jerome once said was a bit like car insurance. It was fine until and unless you claim. I have tried hard to get back into NHS without in anyway trying to jump queues. NHS has the same surgeons, but with a massive support structure behind it too. It was of course fantastic.

Insurers have refused cover on several occasions, including spinal procedures, specific consultants and more recently Sacral Nerve Stimulator. The letters and phone calls have gone back and forth.

August 2018 from insurers

...... as a caring company, we make an exception to cover a sacral nerve stimulator, or in your case a replacement lead, even though this goes against our policy rules. Unfortunately, we cannot provide cover indefinitely so, following the lead replacement, we then advise that no further cover for the entire condition will be provided once two months have passed.

The condition stated was Urinary Incontinence.

As I do not have incontinence I was not overly concerned. Indeed the SNS helps me use my bladder to make me continent!

The Sacral Nerve Stimulator was like a heart pacemaker. It was about functionality to empty the bladder which along with Clean Intermittent Self Catheterisation (which I had not ever asked them to cover) was not only efficient economic and the NICE Gold standard.

Insurers wrote to me again in response to the need for a SNS battery change. Obviously, batteries are not infinite in life. Indeed, new battery technology improves and enhances the functionality of the device. The additional point was that it would enable MRI scanning. If necessary, an MRI for any body part could then be undertaken. It would be a good preventative measure to save any unexpected medical incidents. Obviously saving insurance costs.

An improved SNS would be an excellent cost saving. But they chose to ignore the specialist consultant's opinion and chose to decide this: The *diagnosis as confirmed your consultant was poor bladder emptying and stress incontinence, this was urinary incontinence and all related symptoms. While we understand that ongoing treatment was necessary, the condition falls under and was subject to the terms for a chronic condition.*

I do not have stress incontinence. I have good bladder emptying using the strategies and techniques advised by NICE guidelines and of course my consultants and specialist nurses i.e. renowned experts in this field. In addition, it is the gold standard under Nice guidelines.

> *InterStim Therapy for Urinary Control is indicated for the treatment of urinary retention and the symptoms of overactive bladder, including urinary urge incontinence and significant symptoms of urgency-frequency alone or in combination, in patients who have failed or could not tolerate more conservative treatments.*[37]

---

[37] Medtronic Sacral Nerve Stimulator: https://bit.ly/31p6M7L.

Insurers then wrote to me again.

Following a further letter from your consultant regarding your claim unfortunately the information received does not change the decision on the claim.

There was no further benefit for urinary incontinence and all related symptoms including any complications arising from the implantation of the stimulator, it's maintenance, replacement or removal. This covers bladder dysfunction, repeat cystoscopies, sepsis, recurrent infections, voiding and emptying issues as these are all related to urinary incontinence and the implantation of the stimulator.

It was a longer list of exclusions than before and a diagnosis which was simply not true. The addition to the trying to encapsulate any symptom complication or frankly any part of bladder emptying. As everyone has a bladder which needs emptying this list now becomes totally ridiculous. It would be like telling a heart pacemaker patient that their battery would not be replaced. It would be like telling a respiratory patient that they could not use an inhaler to help them breathe. That was illogical and makes your company sound uncaring at worst, ill-informed at best. Continuity of care does not match the premium we pay for your services. Indeed, I am not sure what you are able to cover any more. How can some anonymous person, who I have never met, who has never examined me nor seen any of my procedures, tests nor results, overrule the Consultants who look after me? The area of private insurance needs addressing.

The situation was perhaps best summed up by Jerome who likens the situation to car insurance. Almost as though the driver was covered, if it was not a Bentley that crashes into the insured car. In which case no cover was available....

Dear Driver,

It has come to our attention that you have recently claimed for an accident. Obviously, this will be covered by your expensive insurance premium that you hold with us.

Our records show that, as you pulled away from green traffic lights, you were struck by a white van speeding through a red light from the Left hand side. This sounds most unfortunate and we hope you are recovering from the shock.

However, although this accident was clearly not your fault, and despite having taken out insurance to cover all eventualities, we need to make you aware of the implications this will have for your policy.

First of all, we will need to put up the cost of your insurance premium.

Secondly, you should be aware that the policy will no longer cover accidents at traffic lights, regardless of the circumstances. Similarly, incidents at roundabouts, T junctions, crossroads or any other form of interception of roads will no longer be covered.

Please get in contact with any queries regarding your ongoing comprehensive car insurance with *us*.

If I have learnt anything it is that shit happens, don't look back in anger, do something to help others. Indeed, my advice was always…get another opinion. Do not ever worry that you are causing offence. It is your body, your life. Just do it.

The next part of the story will have to encompass the very real pandemic that did hit the world. Covid.

What a crock of shite that turned out to be too.

About the Author

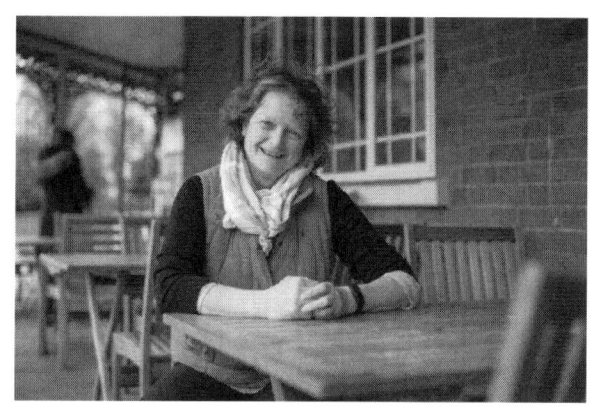

Jacqueline Emkes known as Jacq October 2021

Jacq and her husband live in Bedfordshire. They had previously lived in South London whilst working as Chartered Accountants. Once her four children were at school, she retrained and became a secondary maths teacher.

Since 2009 Jacq has had various urological procedures for complex bladder dysfunction including: boari flap, nephrectomy, colposuspension and autologous rectus fascial colposacropexy. In addition she had to have had stents, nephrostomies and indwelling, suprapubic and disposable catheters too. Infections have been complicated by resistant bacteria and allergic reactions to some antibiotics. The infections have caused rapid spinal degeneration. This led to a spinal fusion in 2011, spinal injections and a spinal implant have been Jacq made the decision to retire from teaching and try to raise awareness of bladder problems. This is a subject that people do not like to discuss. She hopes to break down the taboos. Patients sometimes feel treatments are delivered **to** them rather than **with** them. Patients working **with** researchers and clinicians makes a massive difference to outcomes. d inv

The various groups Jacq has volunteered with include:
- Patient Representative for the National Bladder and Bowel Health Project NHS England and Excellence in Continence Care Board – Chair Patient and Carer forum https://www.england.nhs.uk/author/jacq-emkes/
- Bladder Health UK – Treasurer and Patient Rep Trustee https://bladderhealthuk.org/
- University of Southampton working with Professor Mandy Fader Margaret Macauley advisor for the website known as https://www.continenceproductadvisor.org/
- Attendee at All Parliamentary Political Group (Bladder and Bowel Health) http://www.appgcontinence.org.uk/
- NICE Guidelines CG 171 women's Urinary Incontinence and Pelvic Organ Prolapse.
- https://www.nice.org.uk/guidance/ng123
- Conference speaker at master class events clinical conferences and wherever she can
- Co applicant NIHR project bids
- The Colley Project: dedicated to continence assessment, treatment and management.

- KingEdward7th Hospital Patient Focus Group (London)
- Advisor to BABCON continence app to support people with continence issues by Bristol Health Partners' Bladder and Bowel Confidence Health Integration Team (BABCON), UWE Bristol and associated health partners.
- Patient and Public Voice Partner's (PPV) – Pelvic Floor Health ProgrammePelvic Floor Health Programme. patient representatives to share their perspective and experience as well as champion women and families' viewpoints and voices: <u>Pelvic Floor Oversight Group</u>
- Public committee member on the i4i Product Development Awards Committee NIHR

Printed in Great Britain
by Amazon